Trauma Radiology
Companion

Methods, Guidelines, and Imaging Fundamentals

Trauma Radiology Companion

Methods, Guidelines, and Imaging Fundamentals

Edited by

Eric J. Stern, M.D.
Associate Professor of Radiology and Medicine
Director of Thoracic Imaging
Harborview Medical Center
University of Washington
Seattle, Washington

with

John C. Hunter, M.D.
Frederick A. Mann, M.D.
Anthony J. Wilson, M.B. Ch.B
Wendy A. Cohen, M.D.
Kenneth D. Carpenter, M.D.
Mark S. Frank, M.D.
James P. Earls, M.D.
Lee B. Talner, M.D.
Nilesh H. Patel, M.D.
David H. Lewis, M.D.

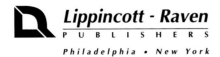

Lippincott - Raven
PUBLISHERS
Philadelphia • New York

Acquisitions Editor: James Ryan
Developmental Editor: Brian Brown
Manufacturing Manager: Dennis Teston
Production Manager: Jodi Borgenicht
Production Editor: Christina Zingone
Cover Designer: Karen K. Quigley
Indexer: Susan Thomas
Compositor: Lippincott–Raven Electronic Production
Printer: Kingsport Press

Printed in the United States of America

9 8 7 6 5 4 3 2 1

Library of Congress Cataloging-in-Publication Data
Trauma radiology companion : methods, guidelines, imaging fundamentals
/ edited by Eric J. Stern ; with John C. Hunter . . . [et al.].
    p.   cm.
  Includes index.
  ISBN 0-397-51733-5
  1. Wounds and injuries—Imaging. 2. Wounds and injuries—Diagnosis.
I. Stern, Eric J.   II. Hunter, John C.
  [DNLM: 1. Wounds and Injuries—radiography.   WO 700 T77627 1997]
  RD93.7.T734   1997
  617.1'0754—dc21
  DNLM/DLC
  for Library of Congress

Care has been taken to confirm the accuracy of the information presented and to describe generally accepted practices. However, the authors, editor, and publisher are not responsible for errors or omissions or for any consequences from application of the information in this book and make no warranty, express or implied, with respect to the contents of the publication.

The authors, editor, and publisher have exerted every effort to ensure that drug selection and dosage set forth in this text are in accordance with current recommendations and practice at the time of publication. However, in view of ongoing research, changes in government regulations, and the constant flow of information relating to drug therapy and drug reactions, the reader is urged to check the package insert for each drug for any change in indications and dosage and for added warnings and precautions. This is particularly important when the recommended agent is a new or infrequently employed drug.

Some drugs and medical devices presented in this publication have Food and Drug Administration (FDA) clearance for limited use in restricted research settings. It is the responsibility of the health care provider to ascertain the FDA status of each drug or device planned for use in their clinical practice.

Contents

Part B: Torso

Part C: Upper Extremity

Part D: Pelvis/Lower Extremity

Contributing Authors

Kenneth D. Carpenter, M.D.
*Assistant Professor of Radiology, Harborview Medical Center, University of
Washington, 325 Ninth Avenue, Box 359728, Seattle, Washington 98104-2499*

Wendy A. Cohen, M.D.
*Associate Professor of Radiology and Neurological Surgery, Director of
Neuroradiology, Harborview Medical Center, University of Washington, 325 Ninth
Avenue, Box 359728, Seattle, Washington 98104-2499*

James P. Earls, M.D.
*Assistant Professor of Radiology, Harborview Medical Center, University of
Washington, 325 Ninth Avenue, Box 359728, Seattle, Washington 98104-2499*

Mark S. Frank, M.D.
*Clinical Associate Professor of Diagnostic Radiology, University of Texas Health
Sciences Center, 7703 Floyd Curl Drive, San Antonio, Texas 78284*

John C. Hunter, M.D.
*Assistant Professor of Radiology and Orthopaedic Surgery, Director of Musculoskeletal
Imaging, Harborview Medical Center, University of Washington, 325 Ninth Avenue,
Box 359728, Seattle, Washington 98104-2499*

David H. Lewis, M.D.
*Assistant Professor of Radiology, Director of Nuclear Medicine, Harborview Medical
Center, University of Washington, 325 Ninth Avenue, Box 359728, Seattle,
Washington 98104-2499*

Frederick A. Mann, M.D.
*Professor of Radiology and Orthopaedics, Director of Emergency Radiology,
Harborview Medical Center, University of Washington, 325 Ninth Avenue, Box
359728, Seattle, Washington 98104-2499*

Nilesh H. Patel, M.D.
*Assistant Professor of Radiology, Director of Angiography and Interventional
Radiology, Harborview Medical Center, University of Washington, 325 Ninth Avenue,
Box 359728, Seattle, Washington 98104-2499*

Eric J. Stern, M.D.
*Associate Professor of Radiology and Medicine, Director of Thoracic Imaging,
Harborview Medical Center, University of Washington, 325 Ninth Avenue,
Box 359728, Seattle, Washington 98104-2499*

Lee B. Talner, M.D.
*Professor and Director of Radiology, Harborview Medical Center, University of
    Washington, 325 Ninth Avenue, Box 359728, Seattle, Washington 98104-2499*

Anthony J. Wilson M.B., Ch.B.
*Professor of Radiology and Orthopaedics, Associate Director of Radiology,
    Harborview Medical Center, University of Washington, 325 Ninth Avenue,
    Box 359728, Seattle, Washington 98104-2499*

Foreword

A critical component of the process of making a successful therapeutic decision about a critically ill or severely injured patient is the rapid acquisition and interpretation of radiographic images. The radiologist can be a full member of a physician's group whose interference in critcial illness can decrease mortality and diminish morbidity. But sometimes missing is the insight required to properly conduct and interpret imaging examinations in the trauma setting.

This book illustrates and underscores how radiologists can contribute to the improvement of patient outcome. The contents announce the full engagement and partnership of the radiologist into the integrity and urgency of the management of the severely injured patient.

Michael K. Copass, M.D.

Preface

Harborview Medical Center is the only Level 1 Trauma center for 25% of the geographical area of the United States, inclusive of Washington, Alaska, Montana, and Idaho, and is one of three main teaching hospitals of the University of Washington School of Medicine. Our unique position as the only Level 1 Trauma center for such a large area of the country provides us, the radiologists that staff this marvelous facility, with a wealth of experience and diversity of case material that is unparalleled in the field of trauma imaging. Our patient population runs the gamut from the inner-city knife and gun club, to interstate high-speed motor vehicle accidents, to farming and industrial accidents, to logging injuries, and even to military-related injuries. We therefore highlight the severely traumatized patient, including blunt, penetrating, and multiple trauma cases. The material in this book reflects the belief that improved timeliness and accuracy of clinical diagnosis lead to improved clinical management and better patient outcomes. To keep the focus of this book narrow, we purposely chose not to include non-traumatic emergent scenarios.

This book serves primarily as an educational resource to the important clinical and radiological questions that must be answered in trauma victims; the what, when, and how of imaging and the pitfalls to avoid. Our aim in writing this book was to create a comprehensive yet manageable textbook of trauma radiology inclusive of many typical radiographic images. We discuss key facts pertaining to imaging, basic interpretation, and pitfalls of imaging. Since radiologic imaging of the traumatized patient involves the use of all imaging modalities at the radiologist's disposal, we have tried to incorporate the appropriate modalities that highlight the key imaging features of the many injuries discussed in this book. In addition to conventional radiography, we have included many examples of CT scanning and use of CT reformations, angiography and interventional radiology, and even nuclear medicine.

One of the unique portions of this book is a review of radiographic techniques. Although radiographic techniques are of most immediate use to radiologic technologists, they can be helpful for physicians to understand, and for recommending or obtaining additional views. In addition, this book gives a general overview of trauma in our society, a review of trauma scoring systems, and even medico-legal aspects of trauma imaging for the radiologist.

The intended audience for this book includes radiologists, emergency medicine physicians, trauma surgeons, and other emergency department care providers (nurses, physicians assistants, etc.) who need a quick, but thorough, overview of imaging of the physically traumatized patient. This book is especially useful for the diagnostic radiology and emergency medicine residents taking or about to take night call responsibilities in areas of trauma and emergency radiology.

Eric J. Stern, M.D.

OVERVIEW OF TRAUMA

Epidemiology of Trauma

WHY WORRY ABOUT TRAUMA?

Trauma is: (1) common, (2) expensive, and (3) poorly understood.

HOW COMMON IS TRAUMA?

Magnitude: Prevalence of trauma as a cause of death is a function of age. All ages: Trauma is the fourth leading cause of death.

- 15–24 years old: 50%
- 25–34 years old: 55%
- 35–44 years old: 25%

HOW EXPENSIVE IS TRAUMA?

Cost of one fatal injury: $425,000 (1986 dollars).

National costs of injury exceed $100 billion per year in which injuries occur. Moreover, aggregate lifetime costs for those injured in 1985 exceeded $160 billion.

Proportion of total medical costs attributable to trauma distributes with injury severity:

- ≈40–60% for mild-moderate
- ≈20–40% for severe
- ≈5–10% for fatal injury

WHAT IS KNOWN ABOUT TRAUMA-RELATED DEATHS?

- Motor vehicle crashes (MVCs) (≈50%)
- Falls (≈10%)
- Homicides (≈20%)
- Burns (≈5%)
- Suicides (≈15%)

MVCs

- ≈50,000 annual deaths and 5 million non-fatal injuries
- Men account for ≈70% trauma deaths
- Only ≈20% of fatalities were using some kind of restraint system
- Blood alcohol concentration (BAC)
  - In 60% of MVCs, BAC ≥ 0.10%
  - BAC ≥ 0.10% in "drinking drivers" involved in MVCs: 16 to 19 years old versus 25 to 45 years old = 38% versus 65%. This suggests that younger drivers are more susceptible (less adapted) to the deleterious judgment and motor-coordination effects of alcohol
- Regional variation—highest risk in South and West (Alaska, Mississippi, New Mexico, South Carolina, Alabama)

- Seasonal variation is small

Summer	≈30%
Fall	≈25%
Spring	≈25%
Winter	≈20%

- Day of week and time of day variations
  - Monday–Thursday, daytime fatalities higher
  - Friday–Sunday, nighttime fatalities higher

HOMICIDES

- ≈20,000 annual deaths (1986)
- Firearms used in 65% (85% handguns)
- Socioeconomic and cultural variance (Table 1)

Table 1

Blacks:	29.9/100,00
Black men (25–29 years old)	99.8/100,000
Whites:	5.6/100,000
All other:	7.2/100,000

SUICIDES

- ≈30,000 annual deaths
- 15- to 44-year-olds are the largest group
- ≈70% of suicides are white males

WHAT CAN WE DO?

Injury Control Strategies:

- Education-Persuasion (least effective)
- Driver education (75% reduction in deaths of 16 to 17-year-old drivers would reduce national fatalities by 600 to 700)
- Legal Prescriptions: enforcement, penalties and personal myths
  - Helmets
  - Speed limits
  - Drinking and driving
  - Automatic protection (most effective)
  - Crash avoidance (tail lights, glare, braking systems)
  - Injury severity reduction (restraints and energy absorption)
  - Post-crash (fire)

The Radiologist's Role in the Emergency Trauma Center

Facilitate triage! Most emergency department's patient volumes are either feast or famine. When busy, the Emergency Department (ED) is no place for Oslerian evaluation, erudite reviews, or probabilistic interpretation. Opinion should be rendered as discreet diagnoses, or when uncertainty exists, recommendations for further evaluation.

Emergency wards are principally "triage" centers. Provisional treatment is commonly initiated, but it is not the primary role.

The role of an urban emergency department is half walk-in clinic and half of its intended mission. As a walk-in clinic, the ED has controversial, social, medical, and financial consequences, all of which typically occur in facilities that are under-built and under-staffed for the function.

Nonetheless, these walk-in patients constitute a large patient volume, many of whom have relatively long ED stays for observation (including various forms of intoxication).

Particularly when busy (typically not usual hospital hours), facility throughout stresses the physical plant and personnel resources. At peak volume, timely evaluation and treatment in significantly ill patients requires rapid assessment and adept radiologic interpretation.

Emergency departments have a relatively high staff-to-bed (full-time equivalent: bed) ratios, high facilities cost per square foot (third only to the operating theaters and diagnostic radiology), but have a relatively low cost per patient seen ratio.

When the emergency department is in the triage mode (high volume—particularly at night, on weekends, and holidays), radiology must "ramp up" in total efficiency to quickly obtain images, facilitate their interpretation and get this information to the treating caregivers in a "just in time" fashion. The most important decision is whether or not the study is "normal," or requires further urgent evaluation. Speed in provisional diagnosis reporting is more important than the elapsed time until the final report reaches the medical record.

Become a member of the team—not an impartial and impersonal "machine" that provides the caregiver with simple radiologic data. Synthesis of clinical and radiographic data is not only helpful, but strategic. In almost no other environment is the art of consultation (our greatest contribution to general medical practice) so greatly useful.

Your practice should be "hassle free." Take the information to the clinicians, rather than waiting for them to come to get it. Do not wait for them to seek you out, particularly for abnormal examinations.

Tailor your services to the style of practice of your emergency department. Don't just ask what they want, study it long enough to determine what they need. Anticipate the market.

Bragg's law: Interpretative accuracy is a given. You must be accessible, approachable, accountable, supportive—and entertaining. This will generate success.

COMMUNICATIONS:

All abnormalities are communicated both verbally and in our "official" transcribed report. We take particular care to document in our dictated report when and with whom we communicated. When errors are discovered, we notify the appropriate clinicians, add an addendum to our original report, and log the details of the error into a Quality Assurance log book (which we call the "Sheet of Shame"). The consequences of these errors are assessed and documented by the clinician services directly involved in the patient's care, and are based upon review of medical records and re-examination of the patients when indicated.

Blunt Trauma Resuscitation Imaging: The Radiologic ABC's

General Goal: Detect correctable causes of hypotension and hypoxemia. Harborview Medical Center initial imaging protocol includes portable x-rays:

- Supine anteroposterior (AP) chest (CXR)
- Supine anteroposterior (AP) pelvis
- Horizontal-beam lateral of the cervical spine (C-SPN)

General approach: ABCs of trauma and emergency imaging parallel those of clinical resuscitation and inspection (Table 2).

Table 2

	Airway	**Breathing**	**Circulation**
X-ray type	CXR	Pelvis	C-SPN
Utility in	ABC	C	AC

AIRWAY

Endotracheal tube (ETT)
Physical examination unreliable in detecting malpositioning (<50%)
>10% ETTs malpositioned on daily CXRs

- Determining tip position
  - Locate carina
  - Trace inferior wall of left main bronchus (LMB) to junction with right main bronchus (RMB)
  - Reference prior radiographs
  - Relative to thoracic vertebrae
  - 95% between T5 and T7; assume T4-5
  - Tip should be 5 to 7 cm above carina when neck is in neutral position.
  - Why? Excursion can be a total of 4 cm: 2 cm deeper with flexion, 2 cm withdrawal with extension.
- Tube and balloon width
  - Tube 1/2 to 3/4 tracheal width, and lie centrally within lumen
  - Balloon width less than 2.8 cm
- Problems
  - Iatrogenic injury
  - Dental trauma
  - Laryngotracheal laceration or perforation
    - Site: piriform fossa or cricothyroid junction

- - Tip oriented to right with pneumomediastinum with subcutaneous emphysema
- Enlarged (>2.8 cm) and prolapsed balloon cuff (<2.0 cm from tube tip) suggests the tube is not in the trachea
- Mediastinitis? Get CT scan of the chest
- Incorrect position: ≈20%
  - RMB (50%)
    - High FiO_2 rapid collapse
    - Hyperexpansion causing pneumothorax complicates 15%
  - Esophageal
    - Gastric dilation
    - Endotracheal tube projected lateral to tracheal wall
  - Airways obstruction
    - Mucus plugging and secretions (loss of cough mechanism)
    - Dental or foreign debris (emergent or urgent bronchoscopy)
  - Sinusitis
    - Mucosal thickening and air-fluid levels seen in ≈50% of patients after 3 days reflects edema and retained secretions, NOT infection
    - <5% develop bacterial sinusitis, thus positive for sinusitis CT scans require bacteriologic confirmation

Tracheostomy Tube
Stoma usually at third tracheal cartilage ring
Head position has little effect on relationship between tip and carina

- Position
  - Tip should be several centimeters above carina (≈1/2 to 2/3 distance between vocal cords [C5-6] and carina)
  - Width 1/2 to 2/3 tracheal diameter
- Problems
  - Tube angulation
    - Posterior tip angulation
      - Partial or complete extubation
        Tracheal tip at or above stomal flange
      - Perforation of posterior tracheal membrane
        Tracheoesophageal or tracheopleural fistula, or mediastinitis (especially if chronic indwelling NG tube); usually occurs within two to four weeks post-tracheostomy
        Caveat: ALL intubated patients have abnormal swallowing, and aspiration pneumonitis needs to be differentiated from fistula
      - Anterior tip angulation is common with low stomal site and increases the risk of innominate artery erosion
  - Subcutaneous emphysema

- Usual after tracheostomy, but should NOT increase over time; if massive, exclude paratracheal tube location
- Tube-related complications
  - Mucosal ulceration and tracheal stenosis are common if cuff >1.5× the tracheal diameter at the level of the clavicular heads
  - Infectious organisms difficult to isolate because of colonization
- Post-extubation complications
  - Stenosis

    Location: 1.5 cm below stoma; 1 to 4 cm long

    Granulomas at tip level, usually anterior wall

    Symptoms unusual unless stenosis >50 to 75%
  - Tracheomalacia

BREATHING

Extra- and intrapulmonary causes of hypoxemia

- Hemo- and pneumothoraces
- Lung parenchyma
  - Traumatic
    - Contusions
    - Lacerations
  - Depressed central nervous system function
    - Aspirations
    - Atelectasis
- Chest wall and diaphragm
  - Flail chest
- Diaphragmatic lacerations (large)

CIRCULATION

Causes of hypotension, usually due to decreased venous return:

- Chest x-ray (CXR)
  - Tension hemo- and pneumothoraces
  - Tension pericardium (rare, especially in adults)
  - Massive hemothorax
  - Mediastianl hematoma (traumatic aortic laceration)
- Pelvis x-ray
  - Fractures of the pelvic ring
    - Lifesaving
      - Patterns that increase potential intra-pelvic volume (open-book)
      - Patterns associated with major arterial lacerations (vertical shear, involvement of sciatic notch)

- Any pelvic ring fracture can be associated with bleeding; therefore, persistent blood replacement requirements should lead to pelvic angiography and embolization
- Cervical spine X-ray (CSPN)
    - Fractures or luxations associated with neurogenic shock (generally those above the sixth thoracic vertebral body)
    - Craniocervical dissociation (atlanto-occipital dissociation)

SUMMARY

You should be able to reliably and immediately identify:

1. Endotracheal tube malpositions
2. Pneumothorax on a supine AP CXR
3. Tension (hemo- and pneumothoraces, pericardium)
4. Potential major diaphragmatic laceration
5. Flail chest
6. Abnormal mediastinum
7. Pelvic ring fractures
8. CSPN fractures and luxations
9. Pulmonary parenchymal diseases of contusion, aspirations, etc.

Patterns of Injury

PRINCIPLES

- The trauma team must minimize the time to definitive diagnosis and treatment of all clinically important injuries.
- Injuries caused by a specific mechanism and magnitude of trauma are rather stereotypical and not random. Statistically associated injuries and traumatizing mechanisms are patterns of injury.
- Knowledge of either the injuring mechanism or of an injury characteristic of a specific mechanism guides the directed search (clinical and imaging) for known associations.
- Directed search for known associations abbreviates time to diagnosis, promotes early stabilization of patient condition, and reduces the often unnecessary use of expensive resources.

Patterns of injury reflect differences in: (1) factors specific to the injured host (e.g., age, sex, anatomy) and (2) mechanism of injury (e.g., stabbing, pedestrian struck by truck).

AGE

- Children and adolescents better withstand impact trauma, but (unlike adults) significant visceral trauma may be present without obvious body wall trauma.

ANATOMY

- Inter-sex differences
- Differential impact resistance of body parts
- Organ fixation
- Underlying disease or substance abuse (e.g., cirrhotic liver is more fragile)

Inter-sex differences:

- Facial fractures: Adjusted for lean body mass, women have more fragile facial bones than men. For a given magnitude of force, women sustain more, and more severe, maxillofacial injuries.
- Prostatism: Elderly men, especially alcoholics, have a ten-fold greater incidence of intraperitoneal bladder rupture than women of the same age.
- Pregnancy

Differential impact resistance:

- First and second rib fractures
  - 30% mortality (autopsy series)
  - 65% intrathoracic injuries
  - 50% cranial injuries
  - 33% intraabdominal injuries

- Sternal fractures
  - Weak association with myocardial contusions, cardiac rupture
  - Thoracolumbar compression fractures
- Scapular fractures
  - 50% ipsilateral rib fractures and pulmonary contusions
  - 25% ipsilateral extremity fractures
  - 20% PTX if ribs also fractured
  - 10% ipsilateral arterial injuries
- Femoral shaft fractures
  - Patellar fractures
  - Internal derangements of knee
  - Femoral neck fractures
- Thoracolumbar flexion-distraction injuries (including Chance -type fractures)
  - 80% intraabdominal injury in children
  - 20% intraabdominal injury in adults
  - 05% aortic injury
- Aorta
  - Ligamentum arteriosum, horizontal, head-on
  - Intercostal arteries, horizontal, side-impact
  - Aortic valve, vertical (fall)
- Organ fixation
  - Retroperitoneal: Ligament of Treitz, ileocecal valve and mesenteric root
    - Shear
    - Fortuitous loop creation (140 mm Hg)

TERMINOLOGY

Internal mechanisms of secondary and tertiary injuries:

- In general, post-traumatic medical/surgical attention is directed at minimizing the extent and severity of internal secondary and tertiary trauma.

- An injury is primary if it represents the direct and initial disruption. Injuries are considered secondary if the initial trauma causes additional injuries. For example, secondary leg ischemia following a primary bullet wound to the popliteal artery, or spinal cord laceration due to a displaced vertebral fracture. A tertiary injury is similarly removed. For example, tertiary leg ischemia follows secondary femoral artery laceration caused by a primary comminuted fracture of the supracondylar femur.

- Although ambiguous, the distinction between external and internal secondary and tertiary injuries is conceptually important. The most effective intervention for primary injuries (either external or internal) is prevention by the individual persons in a potentially injurious event. However, prevention of secondary and tertiary external mechanisms is often a public safety issue (e.g., air bags for head-on and lateral impact motor vehicle collisions), while prevention of internal secondary and tertiary injuries may be pharmacologic or surgical.

Table 3. Examples of common secondary injuries

Shoulder dislocation	→	axillary nerve
Humeral shaft fracture	→	radial nerve
Supracondylar fracture, humerus	→	brachial artery
Hip dislocation, posterior	→	sciatic nerve
Knee dislocation	→	popliteal artery
Fibular neck fracture	→	peroneal nerve

Blunt external mechanisms of injury:
Strains (tensile, shear, and compression forces) causing tissue disruptions include:

- Primary: direct contact injuries (e.g., pedestrian struck by a car bumper, fracturing the leg).
- Secondary: caroming injuries (e.g., pedestrian struck by car is thrown into a telephone pole and fractures ribs).
- Tertiary: strain inducing deceleration and impact among mobile internal organs or with skeletal elements causing permanent deformation, for example, pulmonary or liver lacerations. (e.g., sudden deceleration of torso caused by telephone pole deforms the liver, which ruptures).

COMMON ASSOCIATIONS

Common mechanisms lead to associations. For example:

Maxillofacial fractures	→	Cervical spine injuries, including whiplash
Fractured ribs 6–12	→	Spleen or liver injuries
Anteroposterior compression pelvic ring fracture	→	Intraperitoneal bladder rupture, male urethral "tear"
Lateral compression pelvic ring fracture	→	Extraperitoneal bladder laceration

- Vehicular crashes: Expressway syndrome, highway-speed, head-on crash affecting unrestrained occupants.

Face or scalp lacerations	→	Cranial injuries
Maxillofacial, mandibular fractures	→	C-spine fracture or whiplash

Zone 1 (lower neck, thoracic inlet, and chest) and/or Zone II (thoracoabdominal region from nipples to umbilicus [in men])	→	Torso injuries (50%), fractured ribs, sternum, pulmonary contusion, laceration, cardiac contusion or rupture, aortic laceration, solid organ injury upper abdomen

- Upper extremity fractures
    - Humerus (15%)
    - Forearm (45%)
    - Wrist (25%)
- Fractures of the pelvic ring
    - Hip fracture and/or dislocation (20%)
- Lower extremity fractures
    - Femur (60%)
    - Around knee (20%)
    - Leg (30%)
    - Ankle and/or boot (45%)

- Vehicular crashes: "T-bone." Street or highway-speeds, front-to-side crash affecting unrestrained or restrained occupants in the vehicle sustaining the side impact

Scalp and face lacerations (30%)	→	Cervical spine fractures (10%)
Torso zones I and II (40 to 50%)	→	Fractures of ribs, scapula, clavicle, pulmonary contusions and lacerations, diaphragmatic disruptions, descending aortic lacerations, upper abdominal solid organ injury
Pelvic ring fractures (10 to 15%)	→	Extraperitoneal bladder injury (30%)

- Effects of position: driver versus passenger (unrestrained)

Cranial injuries:	25% versus 15%
Facial fractures:	40% versus 35%
Chest wall fractures:	33% versus 45%
Abdominal injuries:	15% versus 5%
Femur fractures:	40% versus 65%

- Rear-seat passengers do no better (except kids)
    - Unrestrained rear-seat passenger significantly increases risk of injury to front-seat occupants
    - Restraint system associated injuries include:
- Lap-belt
    - Laceration of mesentery
    - Intestinal rupture/laceration

- Aortic lacerations
- "Chance"-type fractures
- Shoulder belt
    - Submarining:
        - Great vessel (including those in neck) intimal injury
        - Cervical spine fractures and/or luxations
    - Compression: rib fractures; upper abdominal solid organ injury
- Air bags
    - Upper extremity fractures
    - Skin abrasions and burns
    - Facial fractures (short passengers and children, especially if in child restraint seats)
- Penetrating (missile) Injuries:
    - Injuring effects of missiles are by:
        - Crush or laceration (low velocity), which is a function of the cross-sectional profile of the missile as it transits the body. The cross-sectional profile is affected by:
            - Yaw and tumbling
            - Precession
            - Nutation
    - Cavitation (track stretch and sudden collapse), which is predominantly a function of:
        - Velocity (high velocity missiles may have a cavity 10 to 14 times the bullet diameter)
        - Tissue elasticity (Lung has great elasticity, bone has almost none)
        - Fragmentation (medium and high velocity) or number of pellets (shot gun)
        - Ballistics: Kinetic energy (KE) of a bullet is a measure of the destructive potential of the missile. Missiles that remain in the body have dissipated all of their KE, and if a missile has not released some of its energy to the external environment (e.g., passed through a wall) the energy has been dissipated within the body

$$KE = 1/2 \ mV^2,$$

where m = weight (mass) of bullet in grains and
    V = velocity of bullet in feet/second.
Low: 1000 ft/sec (Handguns)
Medium: 1000 to 2000 ft/sec
High: 2000 ft/sec

Gunshot Wounds

KEY FACTS

- Gunshot wounds are a disturbingly common phenomenon in urban areas and a major cause of morbidity and mortality in 15- to 24-year-olds. The mortality rate from gunshot wounds has already exceeded that of motor vehicle accidents in several states. If current trends continue, gunshot wound mortality will exceed motor vehicle accident mortality nationally in less than ten years.

- The nature and severity of gunshot injuries is dependent not only on the type of weapon and projectile, but also on local tissue factors and the distance (range) between the weapon and the victim.

- Handguns and rifles usually fire bullets, while shotguns usually fire cartridges filled with multiple pellets. The wounding potential of bullets is quite different from that of shotgun pellets.

- The objectives of imaging are to determine the path of the projectile(s) and to aid in assessing which tissues have been injured and how severely they are injured.

- Initial workup should always include conventional radiographs (two perpendicular views). CT scans are helpful for preoperative planning, when significant tissue damage to the head, neck, or trunk is suspected. CT is rarely necessary in extremity injuries. Angiography is essential whenever vascular injury is suspected.

- Careful evaluation of radiographs and CT images is generally more reliable than clinical evaluation for determining both the direction of projectile travel and the tissue(s) injured.

Gunshot Wounds *(Continued)*

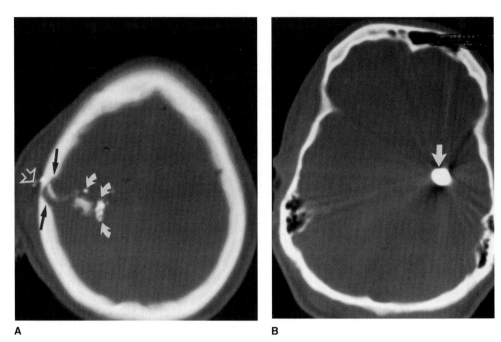

A   **B**

F I G U R E   1   Bullet injury to the head. **(A)** CT scan of the parietal bone shows beveling of the inner table of the skull *(straight arrows),* typical of an entry wound. Note also the bone and bullet fragments *(curved white arrows)* along the bullet track (within the brain), and the outward driven bone fragments *(open white arrow)* within the scalp. **(B)** CT scan from a more inferior level shows the major bullet fragment *(large white arrow)* that has come to rest within the opposite hemisphere. Note that this large fragment can still be accurately localized in spite of the starburst (beam hardening) artifact surrounding it. Because of this artifact, bullet fragments are best seen using images photographed with bone (wide) windows.

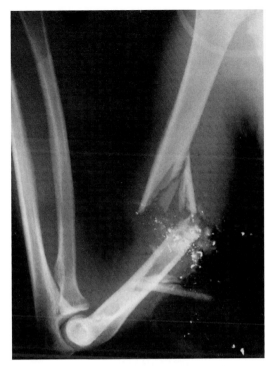

A

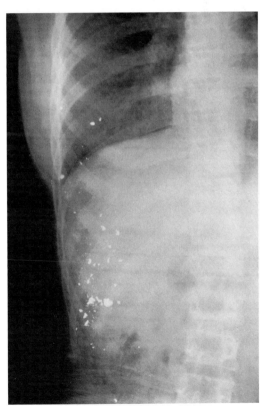

FIGURE 2

High velocity gunshot injury. This patient was shot in the arm by a hunting rifle. **(A)** An arm radiograph shows a shattered mid-humeral shaft and multiple bullet fragments. **(B)** An AP view of the lateral aspect of the lower chest and upper abdomen shows more metal fragments. This patient had a severe liver injury. Note the typical lead snowstorm created by the soft-nosed high velocity bullet. The distribution of bullet and bone fragments shows that the bullet was traveling from lateral to medial.

B

Suggested Reading

Dimaio VJM. In: *Gunshot Wounds: Practical Aspects of Firearms, Ballistics and Forensic Techniques*. Boca Raton, Fla: CRC Press; 1985:99–162, 257–265.

Gunshot Wounds: Low-Velocity Bullet Injury

KEY FACTS

- Low-velocity weapons have lower wounding potential than high-velocity weapons. While close-range injuries with low-velocity bullets can be fatal, medium-and long-range injuries are often superficial.

- The subcutaneous tissue often offers the path of least resistance for small caliber handgun bullets and projectiles from airguns. These projectiles can travel long distances through the subcutaneous tissue, but fail to penetrate the fascia. This is particularly likely at medium to long range, and when the entry wound is at a shallow angle to the skin surface.

- Because these projectiles are sometime a long distance from the entry site, they may not be included in the field of view of the initial radiographs.

- If a low-velocity projectile is not found on initial radiographs and there is no exit wound, additional radiographs over a wider field of view should be obtained.

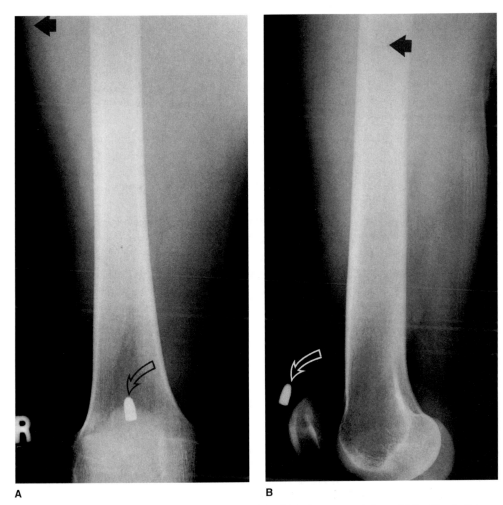

A
B

FIGURE 3   **(A)** AP and **(B)** Lateral views of the thigh shows a nondeformed .22 caliber bullet *(open curved arrows)* lying in the subcutaneous tissue anterior to the patella. The entrance wound *(solid arrows)* was in the proximal thigh. Note that this low-velocity bullet has traveled a long way through the subcutaneous tissue but has not breached bone, joint, muscle, or even the fascia.

Suggested Reading

Dimaio VJM. In: *Gunshot Wounds: Practical Aspects of Firearms, Ballistics and Forensic Techniques*. Boca Raton, Fla: CRC Press; 1985:127–137, 257–265.

Gunshot Wounds: Shotgun Injury

KEY FACTS

- Shotgun injuries differ from bullet wounds. The latter involve a single projectile with each shot, while shotgun shells contain multiple metal pellets.

- While older shotgun pellets were made of lead, EPA regulations now require shotgun pellets to be made of steel. Steel pellets are ferromagnetic and can move, causing additional damage if the patient is exposed to a strong magnetic field. Magnetic resonance imaging may be contraindicated in such patients.

- Steel pellets can usually be distinguished from lead pellets radiographically. Lead shot tends to be deformed by impact with soft tissues and bone. Steel shot will remain round.

- At close range, the combined mass of multiple pellets can produce severe soft tissue and bony injuries. At longer range, shotgun pellets tend to produce superficial injuries that are rarely life threatening.

- As with bullet injuries, the severity of shotgun injuries varies with tissue type and local anatomy. Of particular concern are vascular injuries, as they can result in pellet embolization.

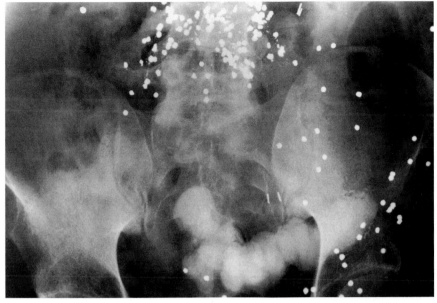

A

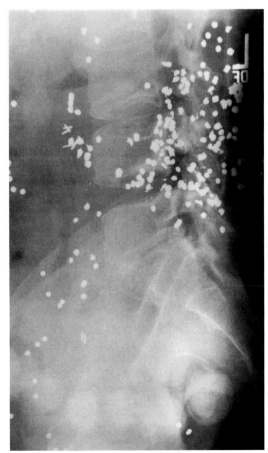

FIGURE 4

(A) AP and **(B)** lateral radiographs of the pelvis shows multiple shotgun pellets posteriorly and on the left. These arose from a single shotgun blast. Deformity of several of the pellets confirms that they are made of lead. *(continued)*

B

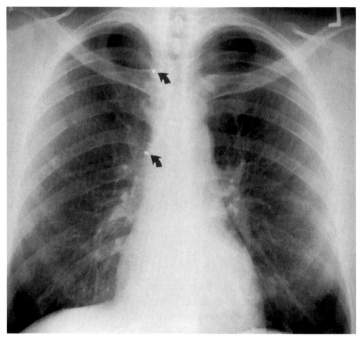

C

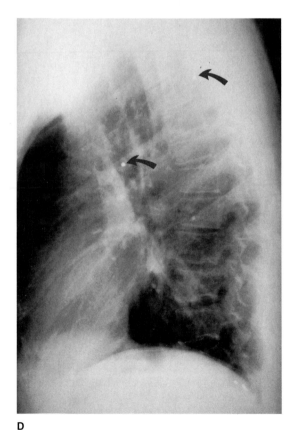

FIGURE 4 (CONTINUED)
(C) PA and (D) lateral chest radiographs
show two pellets in the right lung *(arrows)*.
These pellets have embolized to pulmonary
vessels via the inferior vena. Shotgun
pellets and bullet fragments can embolize
via arteries or veins to a wide variety of
organs. Catastrophic arterial pellet emboli
can occur intracranially following shotgun
wounds to the neck.

D

Suggested Reading

Dimaio VJM. In: *Gunshot Wounds: Practical Aspects of Firearms, Ballistics and Forensic Techniques.* Boca Raton, Fla: CRC Press; 1985:163–226, 257–265.

Trauma Severity Scoring

The severity of a specific injury (e.g., blunt liver laceration) effects prognosis and guides treatments. The consequences of multiple injuries cumulate in a non-arithmetic manner and may result in outcomes worse than those expected from even the most severe local traumas. A variety of trauma severity grading (scoring) schemes are commonly used to estimate the magnitude of individual organ system (e.g., abdomen, head and neck, etc.) and whole body (cumulative) injuries. Scoring systems can direct patient triage to the most appropriate treatment center, enhance prospective recognition of patients at increased risk of death, allow comparison of outcomes between patients of similar injury severity, and promote collection of epidemiologic data.

Trauma Severity Scoring systems are of two broad types: physiologic and anatomic. No current scoring system is optimal for all patient groups, and variation can be considerable among the different systems. In general, systems that aggregate information across multiple organ systems and/or combine physiologic and anatomic data have the best predictive value and the least variance.

PHYSIOLOGIC

Table 4. Glasgow Coma Scale (GCS) for Traumatic Brain Injuries (TBI)

Scalar assessment of eye, verbal, and motor responses

Eye	Normal	4
	To command	3
	To pain	2
	None	1
Verbal:	Oriented	5
	Confused	4
	Meaningless words	3
	Grunts and sounds	2
	None	1
Motor:	To command	6
	Pain localization	5
	Pain withdrawal	4
	Flexion to pain	3
	Extension to pain	2
	None	1
GCS = Eye + Verbal + Motor		
	Normal	15
	Mild impairment	12–14
	Moderate impairment	9–11
	Severe impairment	≤8

Revised Trauma Score (RTS) is based on GCS (above), respiratory rate (RR) and systolic blood pressure (SBP). RTS is a simplification of statistical tools used to predict prognosis following injury, and allow epidemiologic comparisons.

RTS = 0.9368GCS + 0.2908RR + 0.7326SBP; where GCS, SBP, and RR are assigned integer values as shown in Table 1-5.

Table 5

INTEGER VALUE FOR	A GCS OF	A RESPIRATORY RATE OF	A SYSTOLIC BLOOD PRESSURE OF
4	13–15	10–29/min	≥90
3	9–12	>29/min	76–89
2	6–8	6–9/min	50–75
1	4–5	1–5/min	1–49
0	3	0/min	0

RTS ranges 0 to 7.84, with better prognosis associated with higher scores.

For example, a patient with a GCS of 7, RR of 30/min and a SBP of 70 mm Hg has a RTS = 0.9368(2) + 0.2908(3) + 0.7326(2) = 4.2112 RTS and the "probability of survival".

Table 6

RTS	PROBABILITY OF SURVIVAL
1	0.080
2	0.180
3	0.375
4	0.600
5	0.810
6	0.920
	0.970

ANATOMIC

Abbreviated Injury Scale (AIS) is a tabular compilation of hundreds of matched injuries and their code number from the *International Classification of Diseases, 9th revision (ICD-9)*. Injury severity is graded from 1 (minor) to 6 (lethal). AIS ratings can be collated into summary scores (e.g., ISS, TRISS [see below]).

Injury Severity Score (ISS) is a summary score for patients sustaining polytrauma obtained by summing the squares of the three most severe ISS scores from the face, head and neck, chest, abdomen and pelvis, extremities, and integument.

For example, a patient sustaining a subarachnoid hemorrhage (AIS 2), pulmonary laceration (AIS 3) and a comminuted femur fracture (AIS 3) would have an ISS = $(2)^2 + (3)^2 + (3)^2 = 22$.

Table 7

ISS	PROBABILITY OF SURVIVAL (BLUNT TRAUMA)
1–8	0.980
9–15	0.970
16–24	0.875
25–40	0.780
41–49	0.600
50–74	0.340
75	0.150

Combined:

Developed from the Major Trauma Outcome Study data, TRISS is a trauma severity scoring methodology that statistically combines physiologic (RTS) and anatomic (ISS) injury scores, and patient age to provide an estimate of the likelihood of survival for individual patients.

$$P(\text{survival}) = 1/(1 - e^{-b}), \text{ where:}$$

$b = b_0 + b_1(\text{RTS}) + b_2(\text{ISS}) + b_3(\text{Age})$, with Age either 0 (if patient less than 55 years old) or 1 (if patient 55 years old or greater), and

Table 8

	b_0	b_1	b_2	b_3
Blunt trauma	−1.2470	0.9544	−0.0768	−1.9052

For example, a 35-year-old motorcyclist sustaining multiple injuries when ejected into oncoming traffic had an RTS of 4.21 and an ISS of 22.

His probability of survival, $P(\text{survival})$ [i.e., $1/(1 + e^{-b})$], is dependent upon b, and

$$
\begin{aligned}
b &= (-1.2470) + (0.9544)(4.21) + (-0.0768)(22) + (-1.9052)(0) \\
&= (-1.2470) + (4.01917) + (-1.68916) + (0) = 1.08301
\end{aligned}
$$

Then,

$$
\begin{aligned}
P(\text{survival}) &= 1/(1 + e^{-b}) \\
&= 1/(1 + e^{-1.0831}) \\
&= 1/(1 + 0.3386) \\
&= 0.75
\end{aligned}
$$

Similar TRISS regression coefficients (b_i) are available for penetrating trauma.

Medicolegal Aspects in Emergency and Trauma Radiology

Potential issues:

- Consent
- Rapport
- Refractory (belligerent) patient
- Confidentiality

Potential Resources:

- Risk Management
- Social Services
- Courts
- Consultation with colleagues

Consent:

- RBOs: Risks, Benefits, and Options
- Need not provide lesser standard of care
- For incapacitated or unconscious patients, presumption that consent would be granted for indicated treatment (Good Faith and Consultation)
- In doubt?
  - Emergent: time and life running out—treat
  - Urgent: not life threatening, consent from living next of kin

Refusal of diagnosis or treatment:

- Document efforts to explain and persuade, consultation with colleagues and patient family members
- Objecting parent for minor
  - Court order: know how to access court/judge STAT
  - Emergent? Consult and treat
- Abuse
  - APS (Adult Protective Services)
  - CPS (Child Protective Services)
- Mental stability (competency)? Consult psychiatry
- No obligation to put self or staff at risk to provide treatment
  - Aggression control: procedures and training

Reports, records, and documentation:

- Fundamentals: be able to reconstruct care
  - Clear, brief, legible, and honest

- Coordinate care across subspecialties
- Timely
- Date, time, and sign
- Alterations of medical record; must have documentation:
  - Why?
  - Initial and date
  - Caveat: NEVER obliterate original record
- Notifications are usually the burden of the treating caregiver (not the radiologist). Reporting requirements vary by jurisdiction but generally include:
  - Intimate abuse (child, spousal, elderly)
  - Gunshot wounds, stabbings
  - Communicable or contagious disease (e.g., tuberculosis)

Evidence:

- Statements and things that fix facts
- Physical: bullets, knives, drugs
  - Package, label, and give to "proper authorities"
  - Request receipt

Witnessing:

- Percipient (fact) versus expert
- Deposition and discovery
- Your lawyer should
  - Explain case theory
  - Explain what is being sought and why
  - Shape expectations and rehearse
- You should
  - Be professional (candor, confidence, sincerity, interest, calm)
  - Collect thoughts, answers, respond slowly
  - Don't know? Say so
  - Do not argue
  - Strictly answer question asked
  - Do not volunteer information
  - Translate medical argot into lay terms
  - Never say "never," "always"

Malpractice:
"Liability results only when physician fails to exercise the ordinary and reasonable care expected of a prudent physician with his or her special training and knowledge."

- Four components of negligence:
  - Duty,
  - Breech, and
  - Damages with
  - Monetary value
- Notify risk management of potential litigation
- Once enjoined, release or disclose information only after discussion with your attorney
- Caveat: NEVER refer to an incident report in the medical record; it makes the incident report discoverable

Patient Dispositions

What to do about patients with unreliable contact information (address, telephone number, etc.)?

Do what your Social Services recommends.

Try to determine a contact person such as a relative, roommate, or friend.

If a transient, know most commonly used shelters and contact points.

If a life-threatening problem is discovered, notify police agencies (Missing Persons). This may not work in your area, but Social Services at your hospital can be very helpful.

How to handle discordant findings (misses).

We have a daily log in which we write the patient's name, hospital number, exam type, the corrected diagnosis, and then leave fields to be filled in by the Emergency Department personnel for the significance of the error (based on clinical follow-up) and whether or not contact with the patient could be made.

In those cases in which contact could not be made and the significance is considered high, if there was an address available, we send a certified letter to the individual. As noted above, if it is life-threatening, we attempt to contact police for assistance. Again, work through your Social Services.

Methodology must be adapted to your practice.

Comment: This hard copy of misses should be with sufficient demographic information to uniquely identify the case; change in diagnosis must be explicit; and any recommendations must be both verbally and orally transmitted.

Document this exchange of information in the medical record (e.g., as an addendum to your dictated report).

Computed Tomography (CT) Protocols

CT HEAD SCREEN (NON-CONTRAST)

Indications:
   Screen for intracranial hemorrhage, early infarction, dementia or psychiatric work-up, structural abnormality, follow-up head trauma.

Contrast:
   None

Position: Lateral Scout (AP for trauma)
   Parallel to *infraorbital-meatal line* (0°)

Coverage:
   Foramen magnum to top of brain

Collimation/spacing:
   5/5 mm

Photo:
   Standard algorithm
   Soft tissue windows:
      20–40L/250W—through foramen magnum
      20–40L/150W—through base of skull
      20–40L/80W—through brain
      20–40L/100–150W—top cuts
   Blood windows (trauma, R/O any type of intracranial hemorrhage):
      40L/150W (Better if images are a little lighter)
   Bone algorithm-bone windows:
      300–400L/4000W bone windows through base of skull and sinuses

CT HEAD SCREEN (WITHOUT AND WITH CONTRAST)

Indications:
   R/O enhancing mass lesion, AVM, metastases, dural sinus thrombosis. Use when there is also a question of concomitant hemorrhage, abnormal calcification, or of ability to discriminate contrast enhancement.

Contrast:
   Meglumine diatrizoate or iothalamate 280 mgI/ml (2 cc/kg) to max of 150 cc. Use non-ionic if Hx of contrast allergy.

Collimation/spacing:
   5/5 mm

Photo:
   Standard algorithm
   Soft tissue windows: both non-contrast and with-contrast series.
      20–40L/250W—through foramen magnum
      20–40L/150W—through base of skull
      20–40L/80W—through brain
      20–40L/100–150W—top cuts
   Blood windows (trauma, R/O any type of intracranial hemorrhage):
      40L/150–250W (Better if images are a little lighter)
      (Optional 250 width for dural sinus thrombosis, etc.)
      Use non-contrast images

Bone algorithm-bone windows through base of skull and sinuses.
Note: Only need bone windows on contrast scan
300–400L/4000W

CT HEAD—INFANT (< 3 YEARS OLD)

Indication:
Evaluation of hemorrhage. Also, anatomy, intracranial mass lesion, or morphogenesis.
Contrast:
As specified (contrast dose is 2 ml/kg)
Collimation/spacing:
5/5 mm
Photo:
Soft tissue brain
20–40L/100W—posterior fossa
20–40L/80W—through brain
20–40L/150W—top cuts
Blood windows: 40W/150L
Bone windows at base of skull: 300–400L/4000W

CT TEMPORAL BONE HIGH DETAIL (NON-CONTRAST)
Not in the acute trauma setting

Indications:
Evaluation of fractures. Also, cholesteatoma, inflammatory disease, otosclerosis, and implants.
Contrast:
None
Collimation/spacing:
1 mm pitch 1:1 (Helical CT), 1.5/1.5 mm (conventional CT)
Photo:
Bone windows only at 200–400L/4000W

CT FACIAL BONES—TRAUMA

Indications:
Characterization of facial fractures and soft tissue injury
Contrast:
None
Collimation/spacing:
3/3 mm, direct axial and coronal planes
When direct coronals cannot be performed obtain axial cuts with coronal reformats:
1 mm pitch 1.5 (Helical CT), 1.5/1.5 mm (conventional CT). Helical acquisition is preferred
Photo:
Bone windows 200–400L/4000W
Soft tissue windows—30–50L/350W

CT CERVICAL SPINE—TRAUMA

Indications:

Evaluate cervical spine injury. Follow-up of C-spine trauma with *metal screws or plates* **(See NOTE).

Contrast:

None

Position:

Supine—quiet breathing. *Arms pulled down,* if possible, to reduce shoulder artifacts. Check for upper extremity trauma first.

Collimation/spacing:

Odontoid (*from foramen magnum to top C_3*): 1.5/1.5 mm or 1/1 mm

Mid and lower cervical spine (C_3-T_1): 1 mm thick every 2.0 mm (GE helical, *axial* acquisition), 1.5 mm thick every *2.0 mm: Dynamic mode* (conventional CT).

Use a general best angle parallel to intervertebral disks.

Coverage:

Through area of interest. If large area of coverage desired may adjust slices to 3/3 mm. (NEVER use larger than 3/3 mm.)

**NOTE: Be sure the same technique is used throughout the exam or reformats are impossible.

Photo:

Soft tissue windows: 30–80L/400W

Bone windows: 300–400L/2000W (NOTE: 400L/4000W with screws or plates)

Reformats on Bone windows: Coronal (anterior to posterior) and Sagittal (R to L) reformats

Reformats:

Sagittal—All levels: batch from L to R lateral masses 1 pixel thick x 3 mm intervals

For odontoid fractures add coronal reformats through dens

Optional obliques: Approximately. 45° through R and L neural foramina at 3 mm intervals C_3–T_1

CT THORACIC SPINE—TRAUMA

Indications:

R/O Fracture/dislocation. Follow-up trauma post-op with screws or plates.

Contrast:

None

Position: AP & Lateral Scouts

Supine, *arms above head,* if possible, to reduce artifacts, quiet breathing. Check for upper extremity trauma first

Collimation/spacing:

3/3 mm

Use a general best angle parallel to disks through the vertebrae of interest

Photo:

Bone windows: 300–400L/2000W. (400L/4000W with screws or plates)

Soft tissue windows: 30–80L/400W

Reformat:

> Sagittal—batch mode from beyond L to R neural foramina 1 pixel thick at 3 mm intervals
>
> Photo bone windows: 300–400L/2000W

CT LUMBAR SPINE—TRAUMA

Indications:

> R/O fractures, dislocation. Post-op evaluation of Harrington rods or screws.

Contrast:

> None

Position:

> Supine—arms across chest and above area to be scanned, if possible. Check for upper extremity trauma. Quiet breathing.

Collimation/spacing:

> 3/3 mm
>
> Optional 3/5 mm if large area to be scanned (more than 3 vertebrae)
>
> Use a general best angle parallel to disks through the vertebrae of interest.

Photo:

> Bone windows: 300–400L/2000W. (NOTE: 300–400L/4000W with screws, rods or plates)
>
> Soft tissue windows: 30–80L/400W

Reformat:

> Sagittal—batch from beyond R to L neural foramina at 3 mm intervals
>
> Bone windows: 300–400L/2000W

NON-SPIRAL CT ABDOMINAL TRAUMA (UPPER ABDOMEN AND PELVIS)

Oral Contrast:

> If circumstances permit, administer approximately 600–900 ml of water soluble oral contrast material 30 to 45 minutes before scanning, either orally or by nasogastric tube. An additional 300 ml of oral contrast material 15 minutes before scanning is helpful to opacify the stomach and proximal small bowel.

Phase of Respiration:

> Suspended expiration

Thickness/Interval:

> 5×8 mm

IV Contrast:

> Should be used in all patients who have no contraindications to iodinated contrast material.
>
> Total 150 to 180 cc—use NON-IONIC unless reliable history can be obtained from patient regarding contrast sensitivity:
>
> 60 to 90 cc @ 1.5 cc/sec
>
> 90 cc @ 1 cc/sec
>
> 45-sec delay

CT Cystogram:

> If indicated, perform prior to abdominal/pelvic scan—Contrast recipe: 30 cc of 60% contrast added to 500 cc of sterile normal saline.

Instill 100 cc of contrast through Foley Catheter. Quick scan through bladder (spread three cuts over bladder, each cut 5 mm thick) and check images for extravasation.

If initial scan is negative for rupture, continue with additional contrast: fill bladder with bottle hung 30 to 40 cm above table top until filling stops, then scan entire bladder at 5×10 mm to rule out intraperitoneal rupture.

If initial scan is POSITIVE for EXTRA peritoneal rupture, continue with additional contrast, fill up to 300 to 400 cc total; scan bladder at 5×10 mm to rule out intraperitoneal rupture.

Unclamp Foley catheter and proceed with scan of abdomen/pelvis.

Comments:

Pull NG, if present, into esophagus.

If on ventilator, consider possibility of decreasing motion artifact by having respiratory therapy gate ventilator with scan acquisition.

If there is evidence of severe renal trauma, consider delayed scans to evaluate extravasation of urine.

CT ABDOMINAL TRAUMA—PEDIATRIC (ABDOMEN AND PELVIS)

Oral Contrast:

If circumstances permit, administer water soluble oral contrast. Note that NG intubation followed by sedation may be necessary prior to giving oral contrast. Follow approximately the following guidelines:

less than 1 year old: 200 cc 15 to 30 minutes before scan

1 to 5 years old: 400 cc 15 to 30 minutes before scan

more than 5 years old: 400 cc 30 minutes before scan followed by 200 to 400 cc on table

Sedation:

(When necessary) Preferred medication is chloral hydrate via NG tube for infants and toddlers:

less than 1 year old: 50/mg kilogram

greater than 1 year old: 75 mg/kilogram up to maximum of 100 mg/kilogram

Optionally (to accelerate effect) follow immediately with metoclopramide 0.4 mg/kg via NG tube with maximum total dose of 5 mg. If child is too combative for NG intubation, administer IV Nembutal instead:

Maximum of 8 mg/kg; start with 3 mg/kg slow IV push, wait 5 minutes, and titrate accordingly

Phase of Respiration:

If child can cooperate, suspended expiration

Slice Thickness/Interval:

5×5 mm for children; 5×8 for near adult-sized adolescents

IV Contrast:

Should be used in all patients who have no contraindications to iodinated contrast material. Use NON-IONIC contrast. Calculate total dose:

Total dose = weight in kilograms $\times$ 2 cc

Inject the first 85% as fast as IV access allows. Then begin scanning while remaining 15% is being injected

Comments:

Pull NG, if present, into esophagus.

If on ventilator, consider possibility of decreasing motion artifact by having respiratory therapy gate ventilator with scan acquisition.

If there is evidence of severe renal trauma, consider delayed scans to evaluate extravasation of urine.

CT RETROPERITONEUM—R/O RETROPERITONEAL HEMATOMA

Oral Contrast:

600 to 900 ml (roughly two 12-ounce cups) oral contrast material delivered to patient 90 to 120 minutes before the scan. One cup to be consumed immediately, then one cup 60 minutes before scan. Administer an additional cup (300 to 400 ml) oral contrast material immediately before scanning. Use only water soluble contrast if bowel perforation is a diagnostic consideration.

Phase of Respiration:

Suspended expiration

Slice Thickness/Interval:

10×20 mm without contrast, then 5×8 mm with contrast if diagnostic questions remain

IV Contrast:

A contrast scan is necessary if any intrinsic retroperitoneal pathology is questioned. IV contrast may not be necessary if only consideration is to rule out a retroperitoneal hematoma (e.g., from an iatrogenic high femoral artery puncture)

May be used in all patients who have no contraindications to iodinated contrast material. Total 150 to 180 cc: —60 to 90 cc @ 1.5 cc/sec;

90 cc @ 1 cc/sec

45-sec delay

Comments:

If a laceration of the femoral artery is suspected (e.g., from femoral arterial puncture), consider extending scan inferiorly to assess presence of hematoma within the thigh.

CT ABDOMINAL AORTA (R/O ANEURYSM)

Oral Contrast:

600 to 900 ml (roughly two 12-ounce cups) oral contrast material delivered to patient 90 to 120 minutes before the scan. One cup to be consumed immediately, then one cup 60 minutes before scan. Administer an additional cup (300 to 400 ml) oral contrast material immediately before scanning.

Phase of Respiration:

Suspended expiration

Slice Thickness/Interval:

10×10 (or 10×20) without contrast, then . . . 5×8 mm with contrast

Superior Extent:

Diaphragm

Inferior Extent:
Symphysis pubis

IV Contrast:
Rarely needed to document either presence, or extent of aneurysm, or a leak. May be used in patients who have no contraindications to iodinated contrast material. Total 150 to 180 cc:
60 to 90 cc @ 1.5 cc/sec
90 cc @ 1 cc/sec
45-sec delay

Comments:
Pull NG, if present, into esophagus.

If on ventilator, consider possibility of decreasing motion artifact by having respiratory therapy gate ventilator with scan acquisition.

CT CHEST (HEMOPTYSIS PROTOCOL)

Patient Position:
Supine

Proximal/Distal Extent:
Apex lung to lung base, full suspended inspiration in three series:
Series #1: Top of lungs to 20 mm above the trachael carina. 1.5 Collimation with 10 mm spacing.
Series #2: 16 scans from 20 mm above trachael carina to 60 mm below trachael carina (total 80 mm) at 5 mm collimation and 5 mm spacing.
Series #3: From the bottom of Series #2 through to lung bases at 1.5 mm collimation, 10 mm spacing.

Technique:
Bone algorithm; KVP = 120; MA = 170; Scan time = 2 sec; Matrix/FOV = 512/full

Contrast:
150 cc uniphasic @ 1 cc/sec

Photography:
12 on one. Two settings:

1. Mediastinal setting: 20L/450W

2. Lung window: −750L/1500W

CT CHEST—R/O DISSECTION OR ANEURYSM

Oral Contrast:
Usually none

Phase of Respiration:
Suspended Inspiration

Slice Thickness/Interval:
Without contrast: 7 mm 1:1 pitch from 3 to 4 cm above arch downward through thoracic aorta (and abdominal aorta if suspected). Then repeat with contrast.

Superior Extent:
Just above aortic arch (including proximal great vessels).

Inferior Extent:

Through kidneys (or through iliac arteries, if necessary to delineate inferior extent of the dissection of aneurysm).

IV Contrast:

Should be used in all patients who have no contraindications to iodinated contrast material.

Total 150 to 180 cc:

60 to 90 cc @ 1.5 cc/sec

90 cc @ 1 cc/sec

30 to 40-sec delay

Scan downwards

Spiral CT Protocols

CT ABDOMINAL TRAUMA (UPPER ABDOMEN AND PELVIS)

Oral Contrast:

If circumstances permit, administer approximately 600 to 900 ml of water soluble oral contrast material 30 to 45 minutes before scanning, either orally or by nasogastric tube. An additional 300 ml of oral contrast material 15 minutes before scanning is helpful to opacify the stomach and proximal small bowel.

Phase of Respiration:

Suspended inspiration

Slice of Thickness/Interval:

7 mm

Superior Extent:

Diaphragm

Inferior Extent:

Symphysis pubis

IV Contrast:

150 cc @ 2.5 cc/sec, with 60-sec scan delay.

Scan from top of liver to iliac crest.

Wait 2 minutes, then scan pelvis to symphysis pubis or lower if proximal thighs need to be included.

CT Cystogram:

If indicated, perform prior to abdominal/pelvic scan:

Contrast recipe: 30 cc of 60% contrast added to 500 cc of sterile normal saline.

Instill 100 cc of contrast through Foley catheter. Quick scan through bladder (spread three cuts over bladder, each cut 5 mm thick) and check images for extravasation.

If initial scan is negative for rupture, continue with additional contrast: fill bladder with bottle hung 30 to 40 cm above table top until filling stops, then spiral scan entire bladder at 7 mm to rule out intraperitoneal rupture.

If initial scan is POSITIVE for EXTRA peritoneal rupture, continue with additional contrast, fill up to 300 to 400 cc total; spiral scan bladder at 7 mm to rule out intraperitoneal rupture.

Unclamp Foley catheter and proceed with scan of abdomen/pelvis.

Comments:

Pull NG, if present, into esophagus.

If on ventilator, consider possibility of decreasing motion artifact by having respiratory therapy gate ventilator with scan acquisition.

If there is evidence of severe renal trauma, consider delayed scans to evaluate extravasation of urine.

CT ABDOMINAL AORTA (R/O AAA)

Oral Contrast:

600 to 900 ml (roughly two 12-ounce cups) positive oral contrast material delivered to patient 90 to 120 minutes before the scan. One cup to be

consumed immediately, then one cup 60 minutes before scan. Administer an additional cup (300 to 400 ml) oral contrast material immediately before scanning.

Phase of Respiration:

Suspended inspiration

Slice of Thickness/Interval:

Spiral scan:

7 mm spiral with 2:1 pitch without contrast, then . . . 7 mm spiral 1:1 pitch during contrast.

Superior Extent:

Diaphragm

Inferior Extent:

Symphysis pubis

IV Contrast:

Use in patients who have no contraindications to iodinated contrast material. Spiral scan: 150 ml 60% contrast @ 2.5 ml/sec, 60-sec scan delay.

Comments:

Pull NG, if present, into esophagus.

If on ventilator, consider possibility of decreasing motion artifact by having respiratory therapy gate ventilator with scan acquisition.

CT RETROPERITONEUM—R/O RETROPERITONEAL HEMATOMA

Oral Contrast:

600 to 900 ml (roughly two 12-ounce cups) oral contrast material delivered to patient 90 to 120 minutes before the scan. One cup to be consumed immediately, then one cup 60 minutes before scan. Administer an additional cup (300 to 400 ml) oral contrast material immediately before scanning. Use only water soluble contrast if bowel perforation is a diagnostic consideration.

Phase of Respiration:

Spiral: suspended inspiration

Slice Thickness/Interval:

Spiral: 10 mm at 2/1 pitch without contrast, then 7 mm 1/1 pitch with contrast if question remains.

Superior Extent:

Diaphragm

Inferior Extent:

Symphysis pubis

IV Contrast:

A contrast scan is necessary if any intrinsic retroperitoneal pathology is questioned. IV contrast may not be necessary if only consideration is to rule out a retroperitoneal hematoma (e.g., from an iatrogenic high femoral artery puncture). Total 150 to 180 cc: Spiral: 2.5 ml/sec; 60-sec scan delay.

Comments:

If a laceration of the femoral artery is suspected (e.g., from femoral arterial puncture), consider extending scan inferiorly to assess presence of hematoma within the thigh.

NON-CONTRAST HELICAL CT SURVEY ("CT KUB")

Indications:

Acute flank pain, R/O "ureteral colic." Microscopic hematuria usually present.

Protocol:

5 mm slice thickness, @ 1.5:1 pitch, top of kidneys to bottom of bladder (spiral), or contiguous sections @ 5 mm intervals (i.e., no interslice gap).

If clearly positive (i.e., signs of ureteral obstruction and stone in ureter), no further studies needed. Diagnosis of obstructing calculus certain.

If clearly normal (i.e., no kidney asymmetry, no evidence of obstruction and no calcification in the path of the ureter, no further urinary tract studies are needed.

If equivocal (e.g., asymmetric kidney size, or unilateral perinephric stranding, with calcification in the path of the ureter (ureterolith versus phlebolith or iliac artery calcification), or evidence of other renal pathology: give 100 ml contrast material at 1.5 ml per second followed by spiral run (1.5:1.5 mm thick slices, no gap) through the kidneys 5 minutes after end of injection. These images will show whether there is a delayed nephrogram on the side of symptoms and will show other renal pathology (e.g., pyelonephritis, infarct, tumor) if present.

If kidneys appear normal (i.e., symmetric nephrograms and symmetric early excretion of contrast) the study can be ended at this point. If there was a calcification, possibly in the ureter on the CT KUB, consider obtaining delayed CT images at the appropriate level to see if the calcification is inside or outside the ureter. Non-obstructing calculi in the ureter do occur. Actively monitor the study and make decisions along the way. You can substitute overhead radiographs for delayed CT scans.

Almost half the patients with hematuria and flank pain who are sent for imaging actually have an obstructing stone. Most of these will show classic findings on the non-contrast CT, so contrast can be avoided. Contrast should be given when the CT KUB findings are equivocal. In 10 to 25% of patients without an obstructing stone, a non urinary cause of pain will be demonstrated.

CT INTRAVENOUS UROGRAPHY (CT IVU) IN THE EMERGENCY PATIENT

Indications:

Acute, gross hematuria

Pyelonephritis, not improving; R/O obstruction or abscess

Protocol:

KUB before moving patient to CT scanner

Helical 5 mm sections at 1.5 to 1 pitch, pre and 90-second post contrast, through kidneys (film at 7.5 mm intervals)

Patient taken immediately from CT scanner for full abdomen radiograph (5 minutes post-injection film). Subsequent filming tailored to the clinical problem and findings on the early films. For example, if the study is done to exclude abscess or obstruction, you may want to terminate the study right after the 5-minute film if all the questions have been answered.

The usual trauma abdomen/pelvis CT protocol should be used in patients suspected of having renal or ureteral trauma.

Special Procedures in the Emergency Room

URETHROGRAMS WITHOUT FLUOROSCOPY

Standard retrograde urethrogram (RUG): no transurethral catheter in place.

- Supplies: 12 or 14 French Foley with 5 cc balloon; no lubricant (Velcro "choker" or similar tourniquet); 50 cc irrigation syringe; 5 cc Leur-lock syringe; 50 cc 28 to 30% iodine containing ionic contrast (e.g., Conray 60, "full strength" = 28% iodine).
- Patient positioning: oblique or supine (if on a backboard or known to have pelvic fracture). Collimate field to exclude distal-most pendulous urethra and your hands, and center just caudal to symphysis pubis.
- Foley catheter: (1) Before inserting, test balloon using 3 cc air. (2) Fill catheter lumen with contrast (2 to 3 cc). (3) Position catheter through urethral meatus and inflate retention balloon in fossa navicularis with room air until "snug." (4) Alert technologist and gradually inject 30 cc of contrast. (5) Have radiograph exposed during injection when between 25 to 30 cc of contrast have been injected.

Pericatheter retrograde urethrogram (peri-cath RUG): What to do if a Foley catheter has already been placed:

- DO NOT REMOVE TRANSURETHRAL CATHETER!
- Supplies: same as standard RUG, except: use straight catheter (e.g., 8 Fr. pediatric feeding tube).
- Catheter size should be small enough to easily pass along side of in-dwelling catheter. DO NOT USE BALLOON CATHETER!
- Positioning: same as standard RUG.
- Catheter: (1) Fill catheter lumen with contrast (2 to 3 cc). (2) Provisionally place tourniquet. (3) Insert catheter through urethral meatus and position along side of in-dwelling catheter such that its tip is near the junction of the pendulous and bulbous portions of the anterior urethra (in adult, usually 3 in). (4) Secure the tourniquet at the level of the penile corona. (5) Tape catheter to glans. (6) Alert technologist and gradually inject 30 cc of contrast. (7) Have radiograph exposed during injection when between 25 to 30 cc of contrast have been injected *without* contrast spillage from meatus. If spillage occurs, the tourniquet is not tight enough.

CYSTOGRAMS WITHOUT FLUOROSCOPY

In patient with Foley catheter in place.

- Supplies: Cystografin 250 cc, two bottles; hemostats (facilitate removing plastic seals between Foley catheter and drainage tubing); adjustable IV pole.
- Patient positioning: supine. Position central beam to midline at level of anterior inferior iliac spines, and collimate from umbilicus to inferior pubis symphysis.
- Instill contrast under gravity until leakage (intra-peritoneal of any amount or an extra-peritoneal collection larger than 2.0 cm in greatest dimension)

or "complete" filling (>450 cc instilled or intravesical pressure ≥ 40 cm H$_2$0 is the best guarantee that adequate bladder distention has been achieved. Caveat: intravesical pressure >50 cm H$_2$0 may cause injury.

- Obtain films at 50 to 100 cc, 250 cc, 450 to 500 cc, or at whatever instilled volume produces an intravesical pressure of at least 40 cm H$_2$O.

- Notify the patient's nurse of the documented amount of instilled contrast and include this amount in your x-ray report and write it on the film of distended bladder.

- Reconnect Foley catheter to urine drainage catheter and reservoir. Gravity drain the bladder and obtain radiograph with central beam centered in midline 1 in below ASIS (anterior superior iliac spine). [In apparently "negative" studies, this is the MOST IMPORTANT film.]

TRAUMA ESOPHAGRAMS

- For penetrating injuries suspected of transgressing midline structures of the thoracic inlet (Zone 1 of neck and torso) or mediastinum (Zone II of torso). The result of this test is Boolean: leak or no leak. Other than location, characterization is not necessary. Once a leak is demonstrated, the examination is terminated.

- Supplies: Medium diameter (16 to 18F) nasogastric or feeding tube, or equivalent; irrigation syringe 50 cc; 150 cc non-ionic contrast (e.g., Omnipaque 300); 300 cc "thin" barium.

- If patient is unable to cooperate fully, use one of the angiographic suites.

- Patient position: generally, supine; however, prone obliques may be used in cooperative patients. Rotate c-arm to obtain 45° LAO projection.

- Tube positioning, hand injecting contrast and imaging: Position tube tip at junction of middle and distal thirds of esophagus, and position central beam through this point. Collimate vertically.

- Suspend respiration, begin filming at two frames/sec and hand inject 50 cc of the ionic contrast as fast as possible.

- Reposition tub tip to junction of proximal and middle thirds of the esophagus and repeat.

- These two "runs" should image from proximal to distal esophageal sphincters. Occasionally, a third "run" is necessary with the tube tip around T2 level. Injected volume and vigor should be reduced (30 to 40 cc, quickly). If intratracheal aspiration is seen during injection, stop or slow injection.

- Assuming no leak shown, reposition the x-ray tube for an RAO projection and repeat study using the "thin" barium. A final repositioning into LAO projection and "thin" barium sequence is made.

- Reposition or place a nasogastric tube into the stomach and aspirate as much of the contrast as possible.

Contrast Allergy Premedication Protocols

Indication: Patient with prior history of hives, hypotension, laryngospasm, bronchospasm, or anaphylaxis to prior iodinated IV contrast agents. The presence of an anesthesiologist should be strongly considered for any patient with a history of severe pulmonary or cardiac complications secondary to iodinated contrast reactions. In patients with a history of serious iodinated contrast reactions (e.g. anaphylaxis or bronchospasm) an alternative imaging modality (MR) should be considered.

- Prednisone: 50 mg, po, 13, 7, and 1* h prior to study.

  or

- Solumedrol: 50 mg IV, 13 7, and 1* h prior to study.
- Benadryl: 25 to 50 mg PO or IV 1* h prior to CT.

  *This may be given on call for the CT.

If prolonged pre-treatment is not possible, use a single pretreatment at least six hours prior to the study: prednisone 50 mg po or solumedrol 50 mg IV. Then use through a 20-gauge or larger intravenous line.

- Non-ionic contrast medium 2 cc/kg to max of 150 cc (standard dose).

In patients with a history of serious iodinated contrast reactions (e.g., anaphylaxis or bronchospasm) an alternative imaging modality (MR) should be considered.

Minor Allergic History: All patients receiving intravenous contrast should be kept in the department for 30 minutes from the time of injection to monitor for any reactions. In addition, use of non-ionic contrast should be considered if a patient has a history of asthma, hives, or nausea and vomiting, after ingesting shell fish.

Subcutaneous Extravasation During Contrast Injections: The responsible radiologist should take appropriate measures immediately, document the incident in the patient's chart, and convey further therapeutic recommendations directly to the clinician in charge of the patient.

Elevation of the extremity.

Cool or cold compresses for 24 hours. After 24 hours may follow with warm compresses for mild residual symptoms. Full demarcation of the injured site may take several days. If skin injury seems likely, involve plastic surgery and consider admission.

Hyaluronidase: Use of this treatment is controversial. One vial (1 ml, 150 units) subcutaneously per approximately 50 ml of extravasated contrast, injecting evenly throughout the region of extravasation. Use 0.2 ml aliquots and a 25 g needle.

These patients need either a follow-up call by the nurse or radiologist involved in the case or a follow-up visit by the nurse or the radiologist involved. This should be recorded in the chart.

Trauma Radiographic Protocols

Abdomen	Lumbar spine
Acromioclavicular joint	Mandible
Ankle	Nasal bones
Cervical spine	Orbits
Chest	Os calcis
Clavicle	Pelvis
Coccyx	Ribs
Elbow	Sacroiliac joints
Facial bones	Sacrum
Femurs	Scapula
Finger	Shoulder
Foot	Sinuses
Forearm	Sternum and sterno-clavicular joints
Hand	Thoracic spine
Hip	Tibia and fibula
Humerus	Toes
Knee	Wrist

There are two very important facts to remember when x-raying a trauma patient:

1. Work AROUND the patient; DON'T make the patient work around you.

2. Remember the three parallels. No matter what a trauma patient's position, you can get an AP and a lateral of most extremities when the (1) collimator tube, (2) body part, and (3) film are all parallel.

ABDOMEN

Acute abdomen series includes:

1. AP supine and upright abdomen. Label appropriately, 14 × 17.

2. Chest, upright, 14 × 17.

   If the patient cannot stand or sit, a left lateral decubitus (14 × 17) film of the abdomen should be done. The patient should lie with the right side up for 10 minutes before this film is taken. It is important to include the right hemi-diagram, to exclude free air.

ACROMIOCLAVICULAR JOINT

Routine views:

1. AP, upright, bilateral with and without stress on shoulders, if tolerated. Do each side on 8 × 10 or both sides on a single 7 × 17 film. Use 10-pound sandbags. Check the non-stress views for fracture or dislocation, before taking the stress views.

ANKLE

Routine views:

AP lateral, and mortise (15° internal oblique) views. Include the base of the fifth metatarsal on the lateral view. Film size = 10 × 12, AP and mortise on one film.

CERVICAL SPINE

Routine views:

1. A cross-table grid lateral should be obtained first and checked with a physician before moving the patient. If the patient is on a backboard, place a grid cassette at the top of the ear, along the shoulder (at the edge of the board), centering at C4. Shoot film at either 48" or 72" distance. Tape the film in place and have someone pull the arms down.

2. A swimmer's view should be taken if the C7-T1 junction is not visualized on the cross-table lateral. Place a 10 × 12 cassette next to the raised arm, following the body line. The collimator front should be parallel to the film (about 10 to 20° caudad). Use a horizontal beam centered on the ear lobe, cone well, pull down on the other arm, and take on expiration.

3. AP view: use 10 × 12 with grid and angle the tube 20° cephalad.

4. Open mouth view of the odontoid: Place head so that a line between the bottom of the upper teeth and base of the skull is perpendicular to the film. Tilt tube approximately 2° cephalad, cone tightly and shoot through the center of the open mouth.

5. Oblique views should be obtained without moving the patient from the supine position. The tube is positioned above the patient, the beam is angled 45° to the right or left, and a grid cassette is placed flat on the table beside the neck, on the opposite side of the patient. The grid lines must be parallel to the direction of the beam angulation.

Under no circumstances is the head lifted or turned, or the collar removed. The patient's neck should never be flexed or extended by the technologist. Flexion-extension views should be performed only with physician supervision.

CHEST

High KV technique (120 kv):

1. PA, if possible. AP if patient is to be kept supine (e.g., on a backboard). Film size = 14 × 17.

2. Infant or child:

   PA is preferable to AP.

   a. Upright, whenever possible

   b. Do coned down films only

   c. Do not do total body films, unless specifically requested

   d. Use smallest film size possible (8 × 10, 10 × 12, or 11 × 14)

CLAVICLE

Routine views:
AP and 30° up-angled view of the clavicle. 8 × 10.

COCCYX

Routine views:
AP and lateral. AP angle 10° caudad. 8 × 10.

ELBOW

Routine views:
AP, lateral, and radial head views, 8 × 10. If the patient is unable to extend the elbow fully, two AP views must be obtained, one with the humerus flat on the film and one with the forearm flat on the film.

This can be a tricky exam to get on a trauma patient. Remember to work around the patient. If the elbow is bent, place a 10 × 12 cassette between the patient's body and elbow and shoot the lateral view cross-table. The thumb should be turned out as much as possible. The patient should hold his or her breath during the exposure.

FACIAL BONES

Routine views:
Waters, modified Caldwell, and Lateral. The frontal views should be erect and PA, whenever the patient is able to sit or stand. If the patient must remain supine, perform the frontal views AP and the lateral cross-table. The modified Caldwell view should show the floor of the orbit just above the petrous ridge.

If the patient is on a stretcher, all three views are done with 10 × 12 grid cassettes. For AP projections, the cassette should be under the patient's head. If the head cannot be moved, place the cassette under the back board. Angle the tube approximately 15° cephalad for the reverse Waters.

FEMURS

Routine views:
AP and lateral, 7 × 17 or 14 × 17.

The AP should include the hip joint and the lateral should include the knee joint. If necessary, do separate lateral hip and AP knee views on 10 × 12 films.

FINGER

Routine views:
AP, lateral, and oblique. 8 × 10, coned to affected finger.

FOOT

Routine views:
AP, lateral, and oblique. 10 × 12.

FOREARM

Routine views:

AP and lateral to include both the wrist and the elbow. Use the smallest film that will include the entire forearm.

HAND

Routine views:

PA, lateral and oblique. 10×12 or 8×10.

The fingers should be fanned for the lateral and extended for the other two views.

HIP

Routine views:

AP of pelvis. Internally rotate the feet and use a sandbag to hold the feet in position. 14×17.

Frogleg view, with the hip externally rotated and abducted as far as possible. Use a 10×12 cassette. If patient cannot assume this position easily, do a shoot through lateral instead.

Judet views (acetabular fractures):

These are anterior and posterior oblique views of the affected hip region. The patient should be turned and the beam should be perpendicular to the film.

Inlet and outlet views (pelvic ring fractures):

Position the patient as for the AP and angle the beam 30° caudad for one view and 30° cephalad for the other.

HUMERUS

Standard AP and lateral views with neutral rotation should be obtained whenever possible. If the patient cannot move the arm, positioning for true AP and lateral may be difficult. In these cases it is still essential to have two perpendicular views.

KNEE

Four views should be obtained: AP, cross-table lateral (with knee flexed 15°), internal oblique and external oblique. 10×12. Sunrise and intercondylar views should be taken only if requested.

LUMBAR SPINE

AP and lateral. 14×17. Spot lateral of of L5-S1 whenever this area is not well demonstrated.

MANDIBLE

PA, Towne view (centered to the angle of the mandible) and both hemi-obliques. 10×12.

NASAL BONES

Waters view. 10 × 12. One coned down lateral view of the nose. 8 × 10.

ORBITS (SEE FACE/SINUSES)

Waters, modified Caldwell and cross-table lateral views. 10 × 12.

OS CALCIS

Routine views:
Tangential view. 8 × 10. Lateral view. 10 × 12 (include the entire foot).

PELVIS

Routine views:
AP must include entire pelvis. 14 × 17. AP inlet and outlet views, when requested, for suspected fracture of the pelvic ring.

SACROILIAC JOINTS

Routine views:
AP and both obliques, if possible. 10 × 12, oblique position 10° to 20°. X-ray the up side.

SACRUM

Routine views:
AP and lateral. 10 × 12. AP angle 15° cephalad.

SCAPULA

Routine views:
AP and trans-scapular ("Y"). 10 × 12.

SHOULDER

Routine views:
Grashey view, straight AP and axillary views. Trans-scapular ("Y") view should be obtained if the patient is unable to be positioned for the axillary view. 10 × 12.

SINUSES

Routine views:
Caldwell, Waters, and lateral view. 10 × 12. If patient is unable to sit up, the lateral view should be taken cross-table.

STERNUM AND STERNO-CLAVICULAR JOINTS

Routine views:
Lateral and both obliques (PA if possible).

THORACIC SPINE

Routine views:
AP and lateral, 14 × 17. If the T1-T4 area is not well seen on the lateral view, a swimmer s view should be added.

TIBIA AND FIBULA

Routine views:
AP and lateral views to include the ankle and knee joints.
14 × 17 or 7 × 17.

TOES

Routine views:
AP and oblique, lateral, 8 × 10.

WRIST

PA, lateral, oblique and scaphoid views (4 on 1) 8 × 10 or 10 × 12.

IMAGING FUNDAMENTALS

BRAIN AND SPINE

Cerebral Contusion

KEY FACTS

- A cerebral contusion can result from a direct blow to the skull causing inward deformation and brain injury (coup injury). Alternatively, the contusion may result from impacts occurring when brain and skull move at different rates (contre-coup).

- Contusion pathologically consists of small hemorrhagic foci within necrotic brain. On CT scan this appears as areas of mixed low and high density with local edema.

- Contusions commonly involve frontal poles, temporal poles, inferior temporal lobes, and occipital poles.

- Contused brain frequently develops secondary edema.

- Defects from cerebral contusion depend upon anatomic location and extent of injury.

- CT scan is the study of choice. There is little need for MRI on routine radiographs for this diagnosis.

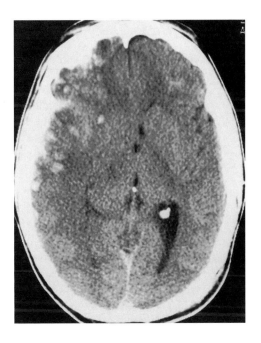

FIGURE 1

Axial CT demonstrating multiple areas of mixed edema and hemorrhage in the right frontal and temporal lobes. There is compression of the right lateral ventricle. This appearance is consistent with cerebral contusion.

Suggested Reading

Johnson MH, Lee HS. Computed tomography of acute cerebral trauma. *Radiol Clin N Am.* 1992;30:352.

Diffuse Axonal Injury

KEY FACTS

- Diffuse axonal injury (DAI), also called white matter shearing injury, is caused by rotational acceleration/deceleration forces applied to brain parenchyma. This causes a stretch injury to the axon. A common cause is a high-speed motor vehicle accident.

- Severity of DAI can be judged by the extent of involvement of more central tissues within the brain. The greater the rotational forces causing injury, the more severe the involvement of callosum and brainstem. Similarly, punctate hemorrhages throughout the brain occur in greater numbers in more severely injured patients.

- Patients with DAI have hemorrhagic and non-hemorrhagic 4 to 5 mm injury foci in the white matter, at the gray/white junction, in the corpus callosum, and in the brainstem.

- There may be diffuse cerebral swelling with obscuration of basal cisterns. There are gradations of severity of DAI both clinically and on imaging studies.

- In general, CT scan will underestimate the extent of parenchymal injury. The extent of brain involvement may be better appreciated with MRI because non-hemorrhagic, as well as hemorrhagic, lesions will be detected.

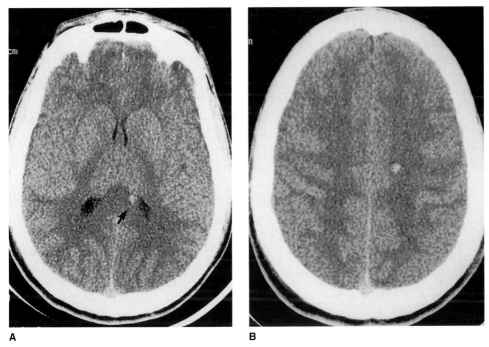

F I G U R E 2 Two axial CT scans showing punctate hemorrhages in a patient who presented with diffuse axonal injury following high-speed motor vehicle accident. The patient was intubated, intermittently comatose, and unable to follow commands. **(A)** CT scan at the level of the lateral ventricles shows punctate hemorrhage in the splenum of the corpus callosum *(arrow)*. **(B)** CT scan at the level of the centrum semiovale shows a punctate hemorrhage at the fronto-parietal gray white junction. Sulci are effaced over the convexities.

Suggested Reading

Gentry LR, Godersky JC, Thompson B, Dunn DV. Prospective comparative study of intermediate-field MR and CT in the evaluation of closed head trauma. *AJNR*. 1988;9:91–100.

Epidural Hematoma/Hyperacute Intracranial Hemorrhage

KEY FACTS

- Patients with acute epidural hematoma (EDH) may present without or with loss of consciousness. Classically the patient has a lucid interval following a blow to the head, followed by an acute deterioration in the level of consciousness. This pattern may be seen 30% of the time and can be masked by the presence of other intracranial injuries.

- Symptoms tend to be caused by the expanding mass of the EDH, especially if there are no other brain injuries. EDH are caused by bleeding from arteries, such as the middle meningeal artery, or from veins. The latter is more common in the posterior fossa.

- On CT scan EDH are biconvex, sharply demarcated, hyperdense collections lying against the calvarium. A skull fractures is associated with the EDH in 85% to 95% of adults and in a lower percentage of children. Often there is minimal injury to the adjacent brain parenchyma.

- EDH may cross the superior sagittal suture or extend above and below the tentorium. EDH do not cross suture lines.

- Signs associated with a poorer prognosis. (1) EDH >2 cm, (2) central mixed densities within the collection suggesting ongoing hemorrhage, (3) midline shift >1.5 cm, (4) brainstem deformity, and (5) extensive associated injury.

- Hyperacute hemorrhages, which are imaged within minutes to hours of initial injury, contain unclotted as well as clotted blood. On CT scan, this is seen as areas of lower density within the clot.

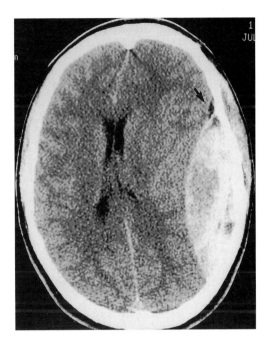

F I G U R E 3

Axial CT scan shows the large left biconvex collection. The gray-white junction is displaced inward and there is a CSF cleft *(arrow)*. The mixed density within the clot is consistent with hyperacute hemorrhage. This appearance may also be seen in a patient with clotting abnormalities.

Suggested Reading

Gean AD. *Imaging of Head Trauma*. New York: Raven Press; 1994:107–124.

Acute Subdural Hematoma

KEY FACTS

- Acute subdural hematoma (SDH) lies superficial to the arachnoid and deep to the dura.

- The etiology is frequently tearing of bridging veins. Another mechanism may be parenchymal contusion with extension into the arachnoid. SDH occurs more commonly after falls and assaults than after high-speed motor vehicle accidents.

- Mortality following an SDH associated with a cerebral contusion is over twice that associated with a simple SDH.

- Acute SDH is seen on CT scan as a crescentic, hyperdense collection, which conforms to the curve of the calvarium.

- Frequently, blood windows (width 150, level 40), as well as brain windows (width 80, level 30), are required to separate an SDH from the calvarium on CT scan.

- Midline shift greater than expected for the size of the SDH suggests associated brain contusion. Shift less than expected suggests the presence of bilateral injury.

- MRI can demonstrate smaller SDH than can be seen with CT scan. This is rarely necessary in the emergent/urgent situation.

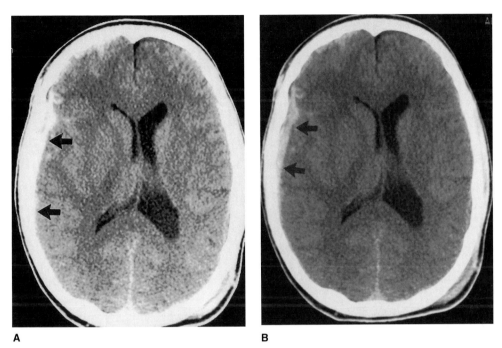

F I G U R E 4   **(A)** CT scan (brain window) showing apparent thickening of the left-sided calvarium *(arrows)*. The cortical densities on the right frontal lobe are consistent with early contusion. **(B)** Axial CT scan using blood windows (150/30) The right SDH is better appreciated *(arrows)* than with brain windows.

Suggested Reading

Gean, AD. *Imaging of Head Trauma*. New York: Raven Press; 1994:78–89.

Chronic Subdural Hematoma/Acute Rehemorrhage

KEY FACTS

- A subdural hematoma (SDH) is considered to be chronic when it has been present more than three weeks and it appears hypodense to brain on CT.

- Peak incidence of chronic subdural hematoma occurs in 60-year-old patients.

- 50% of patients with chronic SDH have either no history of antecedent trauma or a history of minor injury. Other associated acute brain injuries are unusual.

- Postulated pathogenesis includes multiple small episodes of hemorrhage into the subdural space from torn bridging veins, osmotic expansion of an older collection through a tear in the arachnoid, or as a result of protein leaking from neocapillary endothelium of chronic membranes into the subdural space.

- A patient will typically present following minor head injury with mild focal neurolgic deficits or a minimal change in the level of consciousness.

- On CT scan, chronic SDH is a clearly defined, low density extra-axial collection that conforms to the curve of the skull.

- Acute rehemorrhage into a chronic SDH can be seen on CT scan as a hyperdense dependent component within a hypodense subdural collection. Alternatively, the entire SDH can appear isodense when the hemoglobin of the acute bleed is diluted by the fluid of the pre-existing hypodense SDH.

- MRI is more sensitive than CT scan to diagnosis of chronic SDH. MRI rarely is the first ER exam for these patients, however.

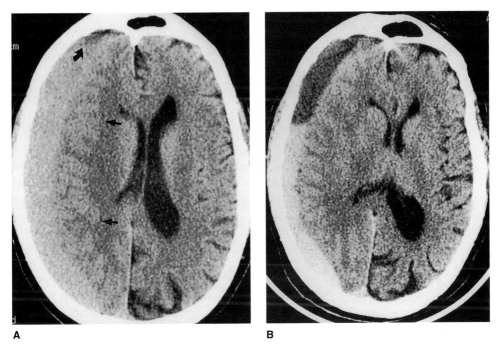

A   **B**

FIGURE 5   **(A)** Axial CT scan in a 73-year-old male shows a large isodense collection on the right. There is buckling of the white matter *(arrows),* compression of the right lateral ventricle, and subfalcine herniation. The subdural hematoma and cerebral cortex are isodense. Note the suggestion of an early fluid/fluid level in the SDH *(curved arrow).* **(B)** Axial CT scan obtained 2 days later shows a clear fluid/fluid level in the subdural collection. With decreased activity on the part of the patient the new clot has settled in a dependent position within the chronic subdural collection. Unlike hyperacute subdural hematomas, the hyperdense portion of the clot is of uniform density.

Suggested Reading

Markwalder TM. Chronic subdural hematomas: A review of 114 cases. *J Neurosurg.* 1981;54: 637–645.

Linear Skull Fracture

KEY FACTS

- Linear skull fractures do not reliably identify patients with intracranial injury following trauma. In adults, 91% of patients with intracranial injuries do not have skull fractures.

- The diagnosis of a linear skull fracture may help distinguish a small epidural hematoma from a subdural hematoma. If cranial traction is required in spinal injury, the location of a fracture may affect placement of stabilization devices.

- Linear skull fractures are often better identified on the CT-scanogram or on a conventional radiograph of the skull.

- Linear skull fractures may not be visible if the axial scanning plane is parallel to the fracture.

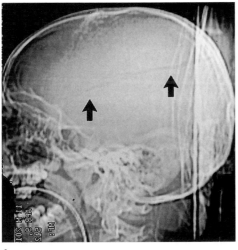

A

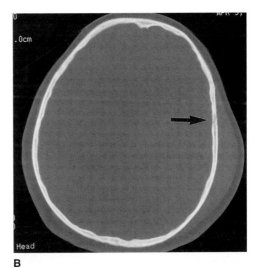

B

FIGURE 6

(A) CT scanogram. **(B)** Axial CT, bone window.
(C) Axial CT brain window obtained in an 11-
year-old male following a fall. The linear skull
fracture, easily seen on the scanogram *(arrows),* is
difficult to identify on the CT bone window
(arrow). Brain windows do not demonstrate
ipsilateral brain injury.

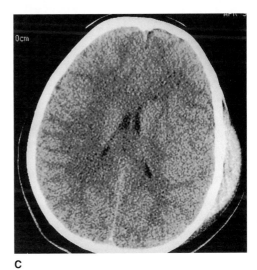

C

Suggested Reading

Masters ST, McClean PM, Arcarese MS et al. Skull x-ray examinations after head trauma. *N
Engl J Med.* 1987;316:84.

Depressed Skull Fracture

KEY FACTS

• Depressed skull fractures are commonly elevated if there is an accompanying open wound, cosmetic deformity, or neurologic deficit.

• The size and extent of deformity of a depressed skull fracture is often better assessed with CT than with conventional radiographs.

• Diagnosis of any fracture with CT is best made using bone windows.

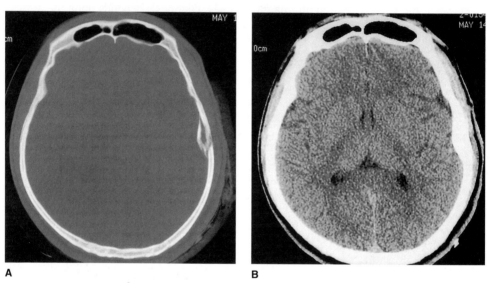

A   **B**

FIGURE 7   Two axial CT sections in a 15-year-old hit by a baseball bat. **(A)** Axial bone window shows clearly the comminuted depressed skull fracture. **(B)** Axial brain window suggests irregularity of the calvarium without demonstrating either the extent or the anatomy of the fracture. There is a minimal underlying punctate hemorrhage.

Suggested Reading

Cooper PR. Skull fracture and traumatic cerebrospinal fluid fistulas. In: Cooper PR, ed. *Head Injury*. 2nd ed. Baltimore: Williams and Wilkins; 1993.

Delayed Posttraumatic Intracranial Hemorrhage

KEY FACTS

- Patients with cerebral contusion or suspected coup/contrecoup injury are at risk for delayed post-traumatic cerebral hemorrhage.

- Most delayed hemorrhage occurs within a few hours of initial injury. Over 80% occur within 48 hours of injury.

- Delayed post-traumatic hemorrhage occurs in brain that previously appeared uninjured on imaging studies. Diagnosis depends upon the imaging demonstration of new hemorrhage without later trauma. Typically this will be on a CT scan.

- Delayed hemorrhage tends to be associated with intracranial pressure >30 mm Hg (normal <10 mm Hg), clinical deterioration of the patient, or failure of the patient to improve.

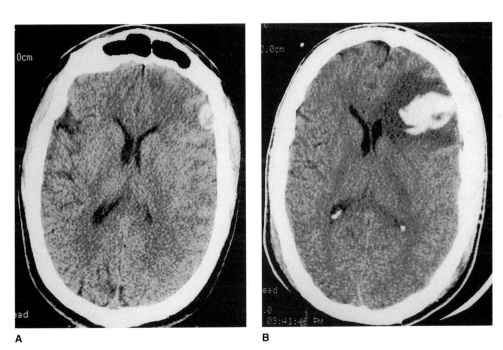

A   **B**

F I G U R E   8   **(A)** Axial CT scan in a 33-year-old male following a motor vehicle accident. There is a small hemorrhagic contusion in the left frontal lobe. Sulci are effaced throughout the left hemisphere without midline shift. **(B)** Axial CT scan at the same level obtained 24 hours later. The clot in the left frontal lobe has markedly increased in size and is surrounded by edema. There is increased compression of the left lateral ventricle. Subfalcine herniation is now present.

Suggested Reading

LeRoux P, Haglund M., Hope A, et al. Delayed traumatic intracranial hemorrhage: An analysis of risk factors. *J Neurosurg.* 1991;74:348.

Child Abuse

K E Y   F A C T S

- 10% of injuries in children under two years of age are due to non-accidental trauma (see Frederick Mann section on Child Abuse).

- Injury typically occurs from shaking the child, which produces a whiplash motion of the child's head on its neck. Retinal hemorrhages are found in 65% to 100% of abused children with head injury. Skull fractures are more common than in non-abused children.

- Diagnosis of child abuse based on cranial abnormalities requires documentation of injury of different ages.

- CT scan of the head is the initial imaging study when a child presents with acute neurologic symptoms. In most cases MRI will better demonstrate the extent of injury and differential ages of injuries; nevertheless, MRI is not recommended in the acute setting as a first study.

- Intracranial injuries commonly seen on CT include subdural hematoma, intracerebral shear injury, or parenchymal hematoma. In these children, it is common for a subdural hematoma to extend into the interhemispheric fissure. (see also acute SDH, intraparenchymal hemorrhage, shear injury).

- Outcome is poor: Mortality is 7% to 30%, severe cognitive or neurologic deficits are 30% to 50%, and 30% will have full recovery.

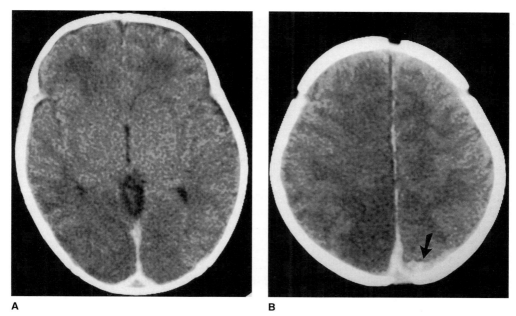

A   **B**

FIGURE 9   **(A)** Axial CT in a 5-month-old boy shows bilateral occipital infarcts, of which the right is more extensive than the left. A subdural hematoma is present within the dura of the falx and sagittal sinus. **(B)** Axial CT more superiorly better shows the thin, left-sided subdural hematoma *(arrow)*. Also apparent is the right posterior circulation infarct. This child presented with seizures. Child abuse was suspected.

Suggested Reading

Merten DF, Carpenter DL. Radiologic imaging of inflicted injury in the Child Abuse Syndrome. *Pediatr Clin North Am*. 1990;34:815–837.

Gunshot Wound to Head

KEY FACTS

- Severity of the intracranial injury from a gunshot wound depends upon the trajectory, velocity, and size of the bullet. Civilian injuries tend to be caused by lower velocity, smaller projectiles than those used in military situations.

- Cerebral contusion and hemorrhage may occur at a distance from the bullet track and are thought to be due to displacement of brain against skull at the time of bullet entry.

- Outcome following a gunshot injury correlates with the level of consciousness at surgery. Mortality in decerebrate patients is 94% to 97%.

- Linear skull fractures are present in 70% of cranial gunshot injuries.

- Extent of the injury is best defined with CT scan. Injury to brain, location of bullet fragments, trajectory of the bullet, and associated fractures can be determined. There is little role for routine radiographs.

- Identification of bullet fragments versus calcium versus hemorrhage may require a combination of window widths and levels: brain (width = 80, level = 30), blood (width = 150, level = 60), and bone (width = 4000, level = 500).

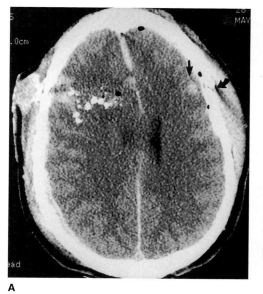

A

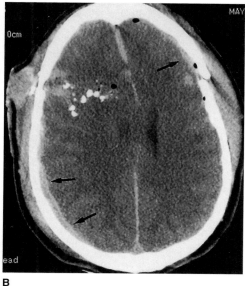

B

FIGURE 10

(A) Axial CT scan (brain window) shows the path of the bullet. There is soft tissue injury in the right scalp at the site of entry. Hemorrhagic contusion, metallic fragments, and air are seen along the bullet track. The falx is bowed. The left brain is also contused *(arrow)*, and there is a left-sided skull fracture *(curved arrow)*. (B) Axial CT (blood window) at the same level better shows the bilateral subdural hematomas *(arrows)* and the left-sided skull fracture. (C) Axial CT (bone window) at the same level better demonstrates the osseous injuries. The inward flaring of the fracture on the right suggests the bullet passed from right-to-left.

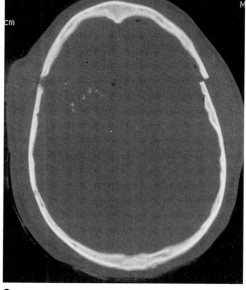

C

Suggested Reading

Nagib MG, Rockswold GL, Sherman RS. Civilian gunshot wounds to the brain: Prognosis and management. *Neurosurg.* 1986;18:533–537.

Cerebral Perfusion SPECT in Traumatic Brain Injury

KEY FACTS

- Blunt and penetrating head trauma strongly affect regional cerebral perfusion.
- Post-traumatic subarachnoid hemorrhage is associated with onset of vasospasm in 25% to 40% of patients.
- Cerebral perfusion SPECT often shows more, larger, and earlier lesions than those seen on CT or MRI after head injury.
- Some of these lesions are contracoup phenomena, while others include diaschisis (functional disconnection of a region of brain distant from a known injury).
- Cerebral SPECT detects the effects of vasospasm on tissue perfusion in patients with subarachnoid hemorrhage.
- Absolute lack of blood flow to a large zone of brain reflects irreversible injury.

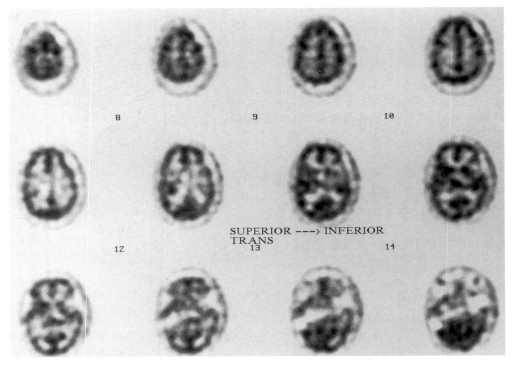

FIGURE 11   Cerebral perfusion transaxial SPECT with Tc-99m exametazime in a patient with gunshot wound to head. Transcranial Doppler showed vasospasm in both middle cerebral artery territories. SPECT exam showed bullet trajectory but no effect of vasospasm on MCA territorial blood flow.

- Hyperemic conditions due to disregulated, increased blood flow after head injury can be shown with SPECT.

- If the patient is injected during a seizure, the scan will usually show increased blood flow at the site responsible for the ictus, therefore, it is important to note the status of the patient at the time of injection.

- After a mild to moderate head injury, a normal SPECT exam is predictive of a good outcome.

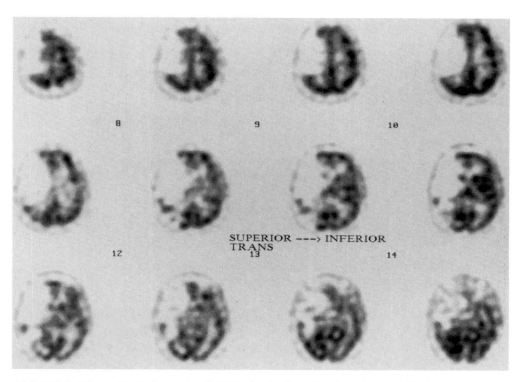

F I G U R E 1 2   Cerebral perfusion SPECT after dural repair and craniotomy following gunshot wound to head. Cerebral angiogram showed right internal carotid artery occlusion. Transaxial SPECT images show severe, large, absolute defect encompassing entire right middle cerebral artery territory.

Suggested Reading

Roper SN, Mena I, King WA, et al. An analysis of cerebral blood flow in acute closed-head injury using Technetium-99m HMPAO SPECT and computed tomography. *J Nucl Med*. 1991;34:1684–1687.

Abdel-Dayem HM, Sadek SA, Kouris K, et al. Changes in cerebral perfusion after acute head injury: Comparison of CT with Tc-99m HM-PAO SPECT. *Radiology*. 1987;165:221–226.

Acute Dissection: Internal Carotid Artery

KEY FACTS

- Acute dissection of an artery occurs when there is a fissure through the wall of the vessel separating intima and a portion of the media from more superficial layers. In the internal carotid artery this can result in a partial or a complete occlusion of the vessel.

- Traumatic dissection of the internal carotid artery is usually the result of a deceleration injury, often associated with other cranial injuries. Deficits following dissection of the carotid artery or vertebral artery reflect ischemic changes in neural structures supplied by the vessel. With carotid artery dissection this includes an incomplete Horner's syndrome and various stroke syndromes. Extensive infarcts occur in less than 8% of patients.

- The mechanism of injury is felt to be a sudden stretching of the artery. This might occur if the neck is hyperextended and flexed to the side opposite the injured vessel.

- Spontaneous dissection of the internal carotid artery may be a manifestation of unrecognized trauma. Less than 10% of patients with carotid artery dissections have disease of the media of the vessel. The majority of patients are between 35 and 45 years and may be hypertensive.

- Diagnosis can be made with catheter angiography, magnetic resonance angiography, or CT angiography. Catheter angiography is currently the gold standard; however, this is an evolving area.

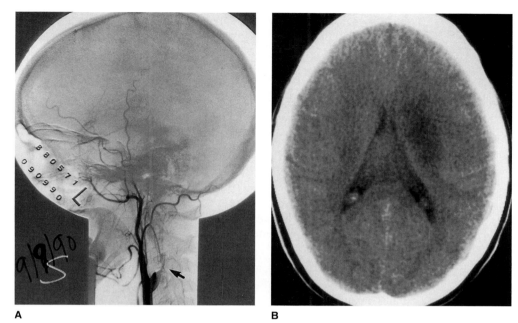

A **B**

FIGURE 13 **(A)** Lateral projection of a left common carotid injection in a 24-year-old woman following a high-speed motor vehicle accident. The patient had right-side arm and leg weakness. The internal carotid demonstrates a rat-tail deformity with distal occlusion *(arrow),* consistent with dissection. **(B)** Axial CT scan in the same patient shows the acute infarct in the left corona radiata.

Suggested Reading

Pearce WH, Whitehill TA. Carotid and vertebral arterial I injuries. *Surg Clin N Am.* 1988;68:705–723.

Acute Intracranial Hemorrhage: Intraventricular Hemorrhage

KEY FACTS

- Intraventricular hemorrhage occurs by contiguous extension from an intracerebral hematoma, shearing of subependymal veins, or reflux of subarachnoid blood via the outlet foramen of the fourth ventricle.
- Possible etiologies of the underlying hemorrhage include trauma, hypertension, vascular malformation, aneurysm, etc. (see subarachnoid hemorrhage, diffuse axonal injury, non-traumatic hemorrhage).
- In trauma, intraventricular hemorrhage is frequently associated with lesions of the corpus callosum, fornix, and septum pellucidum. All of these are found in patients with diffuse head injury. The intraparenchymal injury may not be visible on CT scan.
- Clinical outcome from intraventricular hemorrhage is related to the patient's neurologic status at admission and to the underlying cause of the hemorrhage rather than to the presence of intraventricular blood.
- Hydrocephalus is an unusual complication, found in 12% to 30% of patients. Acutely, obstruction at the outlet foramen, such as the aqueduct of Sylvius, causes the ventricular enlargement.
- On CT scan, intraventricular blood can layer in dependent portions of the ventricle (commonly the occipital horns). Less commonly clot may form a cast of the ventricle.

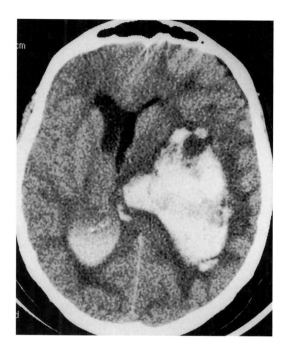

FIGURE 14

Axial CT scan shows a large left basal ganglia hemorrhage that has ruptured into the left atrium. The left lateral ventricle remains compressed and there is subfalcine herniation. The atrium of the right lateral ventricle is dilated and is filled with hyperdense, acute hemorrhage.

Suggested Reading

Christie M, Marks P, Liddington M. Post-traumatic intraventricular haemorrhage: A reappraisal. *Br J Neurosurg*. 1988;2:343–350.

Acute Intracranial Hemorrhage: Subarachnoid Hemorrhage

KEY FACTS

- Etiologies of subarachnoid hemorrhage (SAH) include rupture of intracranial aneurysm, trauma, or bleeding from an arteriovenous malformation. Subarachnoid blood can also be present as a secondary component of intraparenchymal hemorrhage from any source.

- Annual incidence of SAH is approximately 10 per 100,000 people.

- CT scans can be used to diagnose acute SAH. False negative scans occur in less than 10% of patients scanned within 24 hours of ictus. Scan diagnosis of SAH declines with increasing time (in days) from the hemorrhage. Lumbar puncture may be required to exclude the diagnosis of SAH if CT is non-diagnostic.

- The distribution of blood on a CT scan can suggest the location of the aneurysm. Blood in the septum pellucid or interhemispheric fissure suggests an anterior communicating artery aneurysm, blood in a sylvian fissure suggests an aneurysm of the ipsilateral middle cerebral artery or of the carotid artery at the posterior communicating artery origin. Blood in the posterior fossa suggests a posterior circulation aneurysm.

- Aneurysms may be identified, if large, on routine CT scan with intravenous contrast. CT angiography can show 90% of aneurysms >5 mm in diameter as well as identifying the feeding vessel. The definitive diagnosis of intracranial aneurysm currently requires angiography.

- MRI can be used as a screen for unruptured aneurysms. Diagnosis of acute subarachnoid blood can be difficult with MRI. Similarly, obtaining an MRI in an unstable patient following an acute subarachnoid hemorrhage can be difficult.

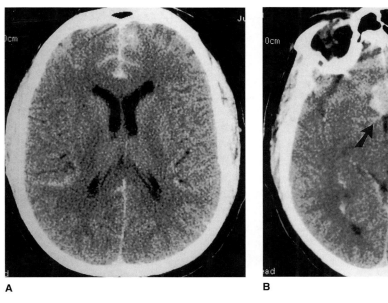

A   B

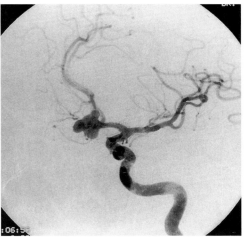

FIGURE 15

(A) Non-contrast axial CT scan shows hyperdense subarachnoid blood in the anterior interhemispheric fissure. **(B)** Axial contrast-enhanced CT scan through the circle of Willis shows the lobulated, enhancing aneurysm arising from the anterior communicating artery. The linear, enhancing A1 segments of the anterior cerebral arteries *(arrows)* lie to each side. Blood is present in the occipital horns of both lateral ventricles. **(C)** Oblique projection from the left internal carotid artery injection shows the lobulated anterior communicating artery aneurysm.

C

Suggested Reading

Silver AT, Pederson ME, Gauti SR. CT of subarachnoid hemorrhage due to ruptured aneurysm. *AJNR*. 1981;2:23–22.

Nontrauma/Nonhemorrhage: Diffuse Anoxic Changes

KEY FACTS

- Diffuse global ischemia occurs when acute cardiovascular insufficiency is severe enough for cerebral blood flow to decline below levels required for cerebral function. A typical cause would be cardiac arrest with secondary prolonged (more than five minutes) cerebral hypoperfusion.

- Within the first 24 hours the gray matter/white matter interfaces may be difficult to identify (loss of gray/white differentiation) on CT scan. This can be seen in the cortex and in the basal ganglia. Diffuse cerebral swelling may not be clearly seen.

- Although the CT scan appearance suggests the possibility of diffuse cerebral ischemia, it does not indicate brain death. Current radiologic identification of brain death requires demonstration of absent intracranial blood flow on a Tc-99 technetium pertechnetate brain scan. Alternatively, diagnosis of brain death is made with electroencephalography.

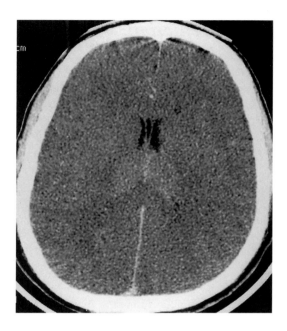

FIGURE 16

Axial CT scan at the level of the lateral ventricles. Cortical gray matter and white matter are the same density, sulci are effaced, and the central ventricles are compressed bilaterally in this patient with diffuse anoxic changes.

Suggested Reading

Kiefer SP, Selman WR, Ratcheson RA. Clinical syndromes in cerebral eschemia. In: Tindall GT, Cooper PR, Barrow DL, eds. *The Practice of Neurosurgery*. Baltimore: Williams and Wilkins; 1996:1775–1788.

Herniation: Uncal

KEY FACTS

- The uncus lies in the medial temporal lobe and forms the lateral margin of the suprasellar cistern. Lying in close relation to the uncus is the third nerve.

- Uncal herniation occurs when a space-occupying mass in the brain causes displacement of the uncus medially. Initially there is compression of the third nerve; later there can be compression of the posterior cerebral artery and the internal carotid artery. When unilateral, the mass is frequently in the temporal lobe. When bilateral, there may be bilateral temporal lobe injury or diffuse cerebral swelling.

- The patient will present with a fixed, dilated pupil ipsilateral to the side of the lesion due to stretching of the ipsilateral oculomotor nerve.

- Other complications of uncal herniation arise from compression of the brainstem and of the ipsilateral posterior cerebral and carotid arteries.

- Choice of imaging modality depends upon the acuity of the presentation. Sudden deterioration in the patient's level of consciousness or suspicion of hemorrhage suggests CT scan. A history of chronic intracranial mass may suggest MRI.

- On axial images, whether CT or MRI, uncal herniation will be noted as medial and downward displacement of the uncus with effacement of the ipsilateral ambient cistern and flattening of the ipsilateral cerebral peduncle. Compression of the contralateral peduncle against the free margin of the falx may occur.

- Subfalcine herniation is also usually present.

- A patient with severe uncal herniation untreated may progress to infarction of the involved hemisphere.

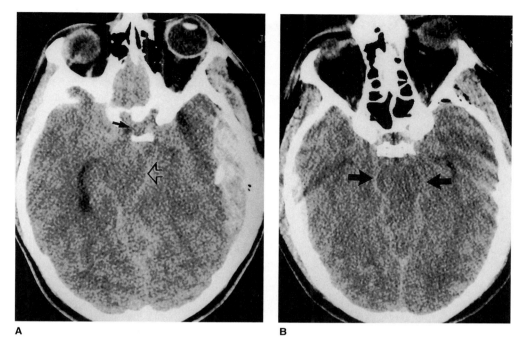

A   **B**

F I G U R E   1 7   **(A)** Axial CT scan through the level of the upper midbrain in a patient with a large
EDH. Uncus is displaced medially *(straight arrow),* basal cisterns are effaced, and the midbrain is flattened
(open arrow). **(B)** CT scan in another patient showing bilateral downward herniation. Basal cisterns are
effaced and the midbrain is compressed *(arrows).*

Suggested Reading
Gean AD. *Imaging of Head Trauma.* New York: Raven Press; 1994:107–124.

Herniation: Subfalcine

KEY FACTS

- Subfalcine herniation occurs when the cingulate sulcus is displaced across midline inferior to the falx and superior to the corpus callosum. Typically, there is a frontal or parietal intracranial mass.

- Similar to other intracranial processes, CT scan is the study of choice if there is acute deterioration in the patient's level of consciousness or if there is a suspicion of intracranial hemorrhage. MRI would be indicated if the history suggested a more indolent process.

- CT demonstration of subfalcine herniation can include shift of the third ventricle, of the anterior cerebral arteries, and of the internal cerebral veins.

- The falx commonly does not shift.

- Infarct from compression of vascular structures is unusual in subfalcine herniation without uncal herniation.

- Treatment of the underlying mass will allow resolution of herniation.

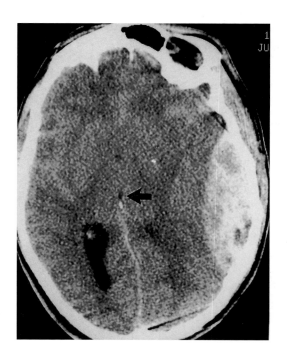

FIGURE 18

Axial CT section obtained more superiorly in the patient with the large left EDH. The posterior third ventricle and pineal are displaced to the right *(arrow)* and the atrium of the right lateral ventricle is enlarged ("trapped").

Suggested Reading

Gean AD. *Imaging of Head Trauma*. New York: Raven Press; 1994:263–267.

Herniation: Upward (Cerebellar Hemorrhage)

KEY FACTS

- Upward herniation occurs when a mass in the posterior fossa displaces the anterior superior vermis upward into the tentorial incisura. Tonsillar herniation can also be present. Acute processes, such as hemorrhage, or a more chronic process, such as a tumor can be causative.

- The common causes of spontaneous, non-traumatic cerebellar hemorrhage include hypertension, vascular malformations, neoplasm, and aneurysm.

- Patients will have signs of brainstem compression, including coma, reactive miotic pupils, and, when more severe, decerebrate posturing.

- CT scan signs of upward herniation include flattening of the quadrigeminal plate cistern with effacement of ambient and superior cerebellar cisterns, compression of the fourth ventricle, increased soft tissues visualized within the tentorial incisura, and hydrocephalus involving the lateral and third ventricles.

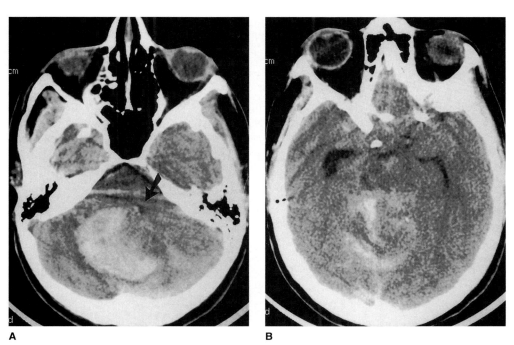

A **B**

FIGURE 19   **(A)** Axial non-contrast CT scan through the middle of the posterior fossa. The large hemorrhage in the vermis and right cerebellar hemisphere displaces the fourth ventricle forward and to the left *(arrow)*. The prepontine and cerebellopontine angle cisterns are compromised. **(B)** Axial CT section obtained more superiorly shows effacement of the quadrigeminal plate cistern and tentorial incisura, flattening of the collicular plate, and dilatation of both temporal horns. This latter finding suggests hydrocephalus.

Suggested Reading
Osborne AG, Heaston DK, Wing SD. Diagnosis of transcending transtentorial herniation. *AJR*. 1978;130:755–760.

Cerebral Blood Flow Imaging for Brain Death

KEY FACTS

- Total lack of brain blood flow, including cerebrum and infratentorial brain, is required for Nuclear Medicine corroboration of brain death in the United States.

- Scans are done by a portable camera at the bedside and include dynamic and static images of the patient's head.

- Use of a cerebral perfusion radiopharmaceutical, such as Tc-99m HMPAO or Tc-99m ECD, is preferred because an agent such as these will cross the blood-brain barrier.

- Other agents, such as Tc-99m DTPA and Tc-99m glucoheptonate, may be used but these tracers require an adequate bolus, proper camera timing, and they do not cross the blood-brain barrier.

- The brain scan can aid in resource utilization and management and the definition of organ donation status.

- The presence of venous sinuses on the images has no impact on interpretation if a cerebral perfusion radiopharmaceutical (HMPAO or ECD) is used.

- For corroboration of the clinical assessment of brain death electro-encephalography may also be used, however, it takes longer to accomplish and "flat-line" readings may be difficult to obtain because of artifacts.

- It is wise to check for interfering medications or conditions that may hamper the neurologic exam for brain death, such as barbiturates and hypothermia, before commencing the radionuclide scan.

- The mechanism for interruption of cerebral blood flow in brain death due to traumatic brain injury usually involves an elevation of intracranial pressure that exceeds cerebral perfusion pressure.

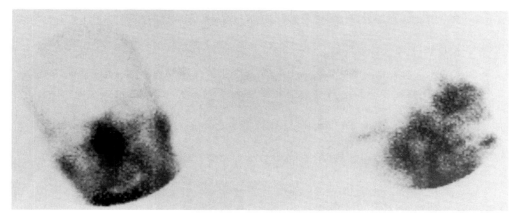

F I G U R E   2 0   Anterior and lateral planar static images of patient with Grade V subarachnoid hemorrhage with Tc-99m exametazime. Images show lack of uptake in brain parenchyma, transverse sinuses are seen in the lateral image. This image shows total lack of cerebral blood flow compatible with brain death.

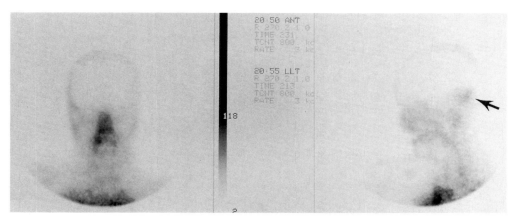

F I G U R E   2 1   Anterior and lateral planar static Tc-99m HMPAO images show presence of uptake in the cerebellum. Although, this is clearly a catastrophic event with no chance of recovery, the presence of some uptake in the posterior fossa *(arrow)* makes this study not compatible with total cessation of all brain blood flow.

Suggested Reading
Reid RH, Gulenchyn KY, Ballinger JR. Clinical use of Technetium-99m HMPAO for determination of brain death. *J Nucl Med*. 1989;30(10):1621–1626.

Facial Trauma: Orbital Floor Fracture

KEY FACTS

- Orbital floor or "blow-out" fractures occur following an acute anterior blow to the orbit. This increases pressures within the orbit, resulting in failure of the thin, poorly supported bone of the orbital floor.

- Complications of orbital blow-out fractures include entrapment of the inferior rectus muscle with limitation of upward gaze, late enophthalmos, and direct injury to the soft tissues of the orbit. If the fracture passes through the infraorbital canal, the patient may have decreased sensation in the ipsilateral midface (V2 distribution).

- Diagnosis of an orbital floor fracture using conventional radiography is best made with either a Waters or a Caldwell projection. Findings may include downward displacement of the orbital floor into the maxillary sinus, orbital emphysema, and air/fluid levels in the adjacent maxillary sinus.

- CT scanning for an orbital floor fracture is usually obtained in order to demonstrate the extent of osseous disruption and to evaluate associated soft tissue involvement of orbital contents.

- Downward herniation of orbital fat may presage late enophthalmos, spicules of bone displaced upward into the medial rectus may correlate to ocular muscle dysfunction. Either a direct coronal scan or coronal reconstructions from thin section axial images are necessary in order to demonstrate displacement of the orbital floor.

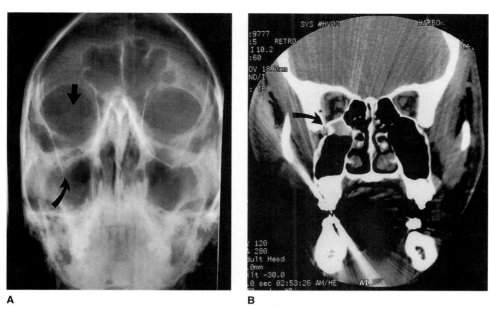

A   **B**

F I G U R E   2 2   **(A)** Water's projection. Patient was hit on the right eye. There is minimal downward displacement of the orbital floor, submucosal hematoma inferior to the right orbital floor *(curved arrow)* and swelling of the right cheek *(straight arrow).* **(B)** Coronal CT shows a portion of the laterally placed right orbital floor fracture *(arrow).* There is associated mucosal edema and fluid in the maxillary sinus. Air/fluid level is reversed because coronal scan was obtained in a hanging head position.

Suggested Reading

Hammerschlag SB, Hughs S, O Reilly GV, Weber AL. Another look at blow-out fractures of the orbit. *AJNR.* 1982;3:331–335.

Facial Trauma: Tripod Fracture

KEY FACTS

- Tripod fractures, also called trimalar or zygomaticomaxillary complex fractures, are complex injuries that involve diastases of the zygomaticofrontal suture (lateral wall of the orbit), and fractures of the zygomatic arch, the posteriolateral wall of the maxillary sinus, and the orbital rim and floor.

- Conventional film diagnosis is made using Caldwell, Waters, lateral and submentovertex projections of the face. However, the full extent of injury, including rotational displacements, is better appreciated using CT scanning.

- Similar to orbital floor fractures (see Orbital Floor Fracture), coronal plane images are necessary to demonstrate disruption of the orbital floor and to confirm the absence of involvement of the pterygoid plates. Zygomatic, maxillary sinus, and lateral orbital wall fractures can be easily identified on both axial and coronal images.

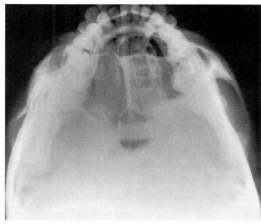

A

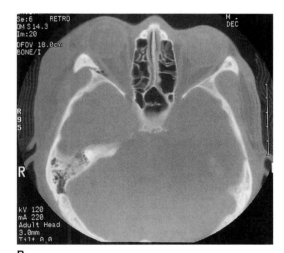

FIGURE 23

(A) Submentovertex projection shows inward displacement of the right zygomatic arch. (B) Axial CT scan through the orbit shows inward displacement of the posterior-lateral wall of the orbit. Intraorbital air probably entered via an orbital floor fracture.

B

Suggested Reading

Gean AD. *Imaging of Head Trauma*. New York: Raven Press; 1994:449–454.

Facial Trauma: LeFort Fracture

KEY FACTS

- Midface fractures are commonly classified as LeFort I, II, or III fractures, or facial smash injuries, depending upon the anatomic region of facial involvement and the complexity of the fracture. All LeFort type injuries include fractures through the pterygoid plates.

- LeFort I fractures reflect dissociation of the lower face from the mid- and upper-face and cranium. Separation in LeFort II fractures occurs at the mid-face. LeFort III fractures encompass complete craniofacial dissociation. Facial smash is a bilateral severely comminuted facial injury with posterior displacement of structures in the mid-face.

- Conventional radiographic diagnosis requires Caldwell, Waters, lateral and possibly submentovertex projections. In particular, the lateral projection facilitates identification of fracture through the pterygoid plates (see Orbit Fracture, Tripod Fracture).

- Similarly to other facial injuries, CT scans are more sensitive to small fractures than are conventional radiographs. CT scan is used to define the extent of injury. Both axial and coronal plane images are necessary. The pterygoid plate injuries and the orbital floor fractures are better appreciated on coronal plane images, whether direct coronal scans or computer-generated coronal reconstructions of axial images.

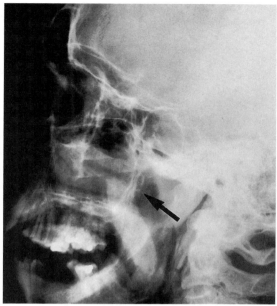

A

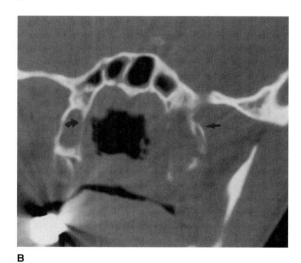

FIGURE 24

(A) Lateral erect radiograph of the face shows fractures of the pterygoid plates *(arrow)*. An air/fluid level is present in the maxillary sinus. **(B)** Coronal CT scan demonstrates a comminuted fracture of the left pterygoid plates *(arrow)* and a non-displaced fracture in the medial right pterygoid plate (curved *arrow)*.

B

Suggested Reading

Gean AD. *Imaging of Head Trauma*. New York: Raven Press; 1994:454–460.

Cervical Spine Injury: Dens Fracture

KEY FACTS

- Fractures of the dens are classified by location according to the scheme of Anderson and d'Alonzo. Type I fractures (rare) involve the tip of the dens, Type II fractures are limited to the base of the dens, and Type III fractures extend into the body of C2.
- Axis fractures comprise 7% to 17% of cervical spine fractures in many series. In one series, 40% of axis fractures were associated with head injury and 18% were associated with other cervical spine injuries.
- Dens fractures are potentially unstable. Symptoms range from pain and neck stiffness to myelopathy.
- Predictors of healing of a dens fracture: displacement of the dens <5 mm, patient age is less than 60 years. Type III fractures have a higher rate of healing than do type II fractures.
- Conventional radiographic diagnosis of a dens fracture requires a good open mouth and a lateral projection of the upper cervical spine. This will show fractures and displacement of the dens.
- If CT scanning is obtained, axial, sagittal, and coronal sections are required to assess the caliber of the ring of C1, the width of the predental space, and associated injuries. Type II fractures which lie in an axial plane, may be inapparent with routine imaging and be visualized only with sagittal or coronal reformations.

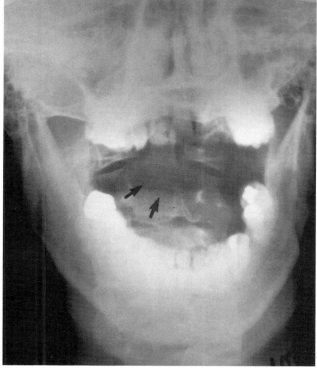

A

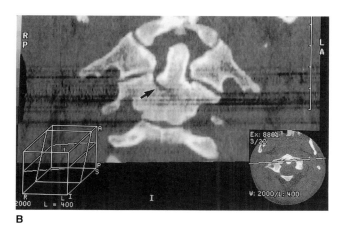

B

FIGURE 25   **(A)** Open-mouth radiograph suggests the presence of a type III fracture *(arrows)* of the dens. **(B)** Coronal reformation from a non-contrast axial CT more clearly demonstrates the type III dens fracture *(arrow).*

Suggested Reading

Hadly MN, Dickman CA, Browner CM, Sonntag VKH. Acute traumatic atlas fractures: Management and long term outcome. *Neurosurgery.* 1988;23:31–35.

Cervical Spine Injury: Jefferson Fracture

KEY FACTS

- Jefferson fracture is a burst fracture of the ring of C1 resulting from an acute axial load. Although originally described as a four-part disruption of the ring of C1, the term is also used for three-part fractures involving the lamina and lateral masses.
- Patients frequently have neck pain without neurologic dysfunction.
- Conventional radiographic diagnosis is best made with an open-mouth view of the upper cervical spine. This demonstrates spreading of the lateral masses of C1. Combined outward spreading of both lateral masses of the dens more than 7 mm on the open-mouth projection suggests injury to the transverse ligament.
- Diagnosis can also be suggested from a lateral radiograph if the fracture through the laminae of C1 are visible. This is a less reliable sign.
- Axial CT scan reliably demonstrates the fractures throughout the ring of C1 and the extent of displacement. Sagittal or coronal reconstructions show associated injury to the dens or to the atlanto-occipital joints, but are less useful in defining the extent of injury to the ring of C1 (see Dens Fracture, AO Injury).

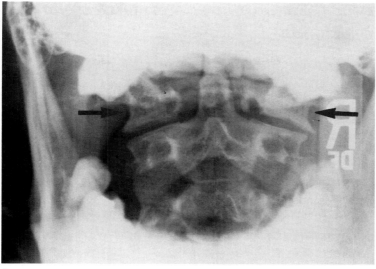

A

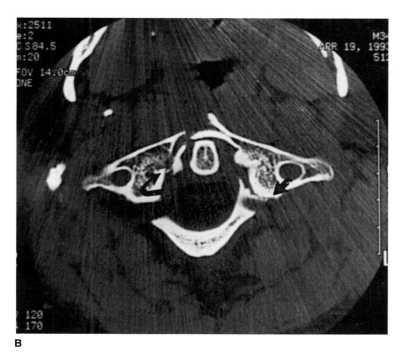

B

F I G U R E 2 6   **(A)** Open-mouth radiograph shows splaying of the lateral masses of C1, more apparent on the right than the left *(arrows)*. **(B)** Axial CT scan through the ring of C1 shows fractures of the anterior ring, right lateral mass (curved *arrow*) and left lamina *(arrow)*.

Suggested Reading

Gehweiler JA, Osborne RL, Becker RF. *The Radiology of Vertebral Trauma*. Philadelphia: WB Saunders; 1980.

Cervical Spine Injury: Atlanto-Occipital Dissociation

KEY FACTS

- Atlanto-occipital dissociation has been described in 8% to 19% of fatal automobile accidents. However, survivors are seen with increasing frequency, probably as a result of improved emergency care in the field.

- Patients who survive may have cranial nerve deficits, quadriparesis, hemiparesis, paraparesis, or lesser degrees of brainstem injury.

- Separation of the cranium in relation to the atlas can occur anteriorly, posteriorly, or longitudinally. Radiologic diagnostic criteria need to evaluate all three possibilities.

- Diagnosis on a lateral radiograph of the head and cervical spine can be difficult because appropriate landmarks must be seen and their relationships appreciated. Plain film diagnosis requires a high index of suspicion.

- Diagnostic criteria on a lateral radiograph as defined by Harris et al:
  - Vertical basion-dens distance ≤12 mm.
  - Basion ≤12 mm anterior or 4 mm posterior to the posterior C2 line.

- Other published criteria, such as the Power's ratio and Lee's X are less reliable than these measurements.

- Diagnosis may be more apparent on sagittal and coronal CT reconstructions than on axial CT images because the displacement occurs in the axial plane.

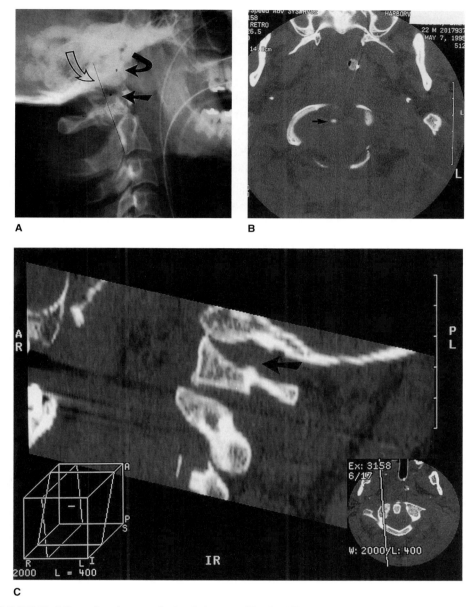

FIGURE 27 Local prevertebral soft tissue swelling is difficult to evaluate in this intubated patient. **(A)** Lateral radiograph showing posterior C2-line *(open arrow)*, top of the dens *(arrow)* and basion *(curved arrow)*. Basion-dens distance is 14 mm. **(B)** Axial CT through the top of the dens *(arrow)*. The absence of occipital condyles in this image suggest widening of the AO joint space. **(C)** Sagittal CT reformation showing widening of the joint space between the occipital condyle and lateral mass of C1 on the left *(arrow)*.

Suggested Reading

Harris JH Jr, Carson GC, Wagner LK, Kerr N. Radiologic diagnosis of traumatic occipitovertebral dissociation: Comparison of three methods of detecting occipitovertebral relationships on lateral radiographs of supine subjects. *AJR*. 1994;162:887–892.

Cervical Spine Injury: Transverse Atlantal Ligament Injury

KEY FACTS

- The transverse atlantal ligament arises off the lateral masses of C1 and maintains the relationship of dens to the anterior ring of C1.
- The majority of patients with injury of the transverse atlantal ligament will have normal neurologic examination.
- Other non-traumatic processes that can affect stability of the transverse atlantal ligament include rheumatoid arthritis, ankylosing spondylitis, and Down's syndrome.
- Using conventional radiographs, the distance between the dorsal surface of the ring of C1 and the anterior surface of the dens (pre-dens interval) should be no more than 2 mm in adults and between 3 and 5 mm in children.
- High resolution CT scan can show instability of the transverse ligament from disruption of its attachment to the ring of C1. Injury to the tissue of the ligament is not seen, although other fractures can be appreciated.
- Injury to the ligament and the joint space anterior to the dens can be appreciated with MRI.

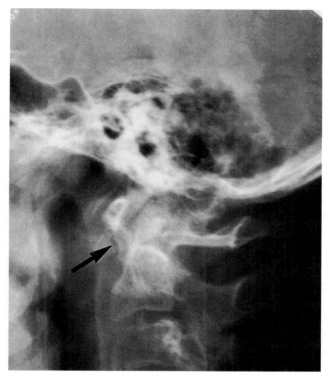

F I G U R E   2 8   Lateral view of the cervical spine shows widening of the predental space *(arrow),* which suggests incompetence of the transverse atlantal ligament.

Suggested Reading

Dickman CA, Grune KA, Sonntag VKH. Injuries involving the transverse atlantal ligament: Classification and treatment guidelines based upon experience with 39 injuries. *Neurosurgery*. 1996;38:44–50.

Cervical Spine Injury: Traumatic Spondylolisthesis of the Axis

KEY FACTS

- Traumatic spondylolisthesis of C2, also known as a Hangman's fracture, is felt to be caused most commonly by acute hyperextention of the head on the neck.

- Neurologic sequelae are uncommon. In general the spinal canal is expanded without injury to spinal cord or nerve roots.

- Fractures are bilateral through the pars intra-articularis of C2. This is the portion of the laminal lying between the articulating facet and the laminar arch. At times the fracture line may be displaced more anteriorly into the vertebral body of C2.

- Diagnosis using conventional radiographs is best made with a lateral projection.

- With CT scan, the fracture may be diagnosed on axial images, but will be better appreciated and understood using sagittal images.

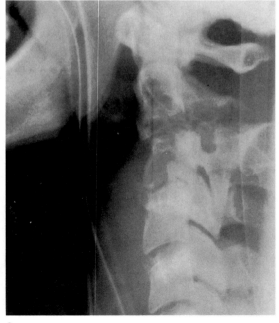

A

FIGURE 29
(A) Lateral radiograph of the cervical spine shows fractures through the pars of C2. The C2-3 disc space is narrowed and the body of C2 is displaced forward. The spinous process of C2 is displaced posteriorly, which widens the spinal canal.

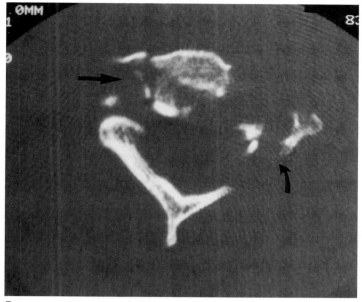

B

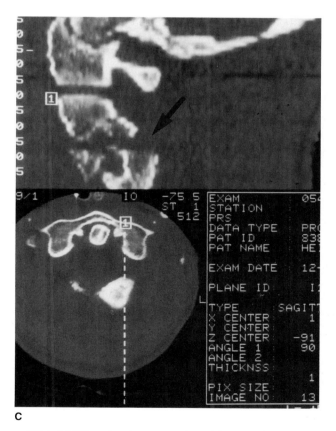

C

F I G U R E 2 9   **(B)** Axial CT section shows comminuted fractures through the right side of the C2 vertebra *(arrow)* and the left C2 pars intraarticularis *(curved arrow)*. **(C)** Sagittal CT reconstruction better demonstrates the fracture through the left pars *(arrow)*.

Suggested Reading

Gehweiler JA Jr, Osborne RL, Jr, Becker RF. *The Radiology of Vertebral Trauma*. Philadelphia: WB Saunders; 1980:171–185.

Cervical Spine Injury: Hyperflexion Fracture/Burst Fracture

KEY FACTS

- Burst fractures occur following a direct axial load on the erect head and spine. In the upper cervical spine this may result in disruption of the ring of C1 (see Jefferson Fracture). In the lower cervical spine the vertebral bodies are comminuted with displacement of bone fragments anteriorly and into the spinal canal.

- Frequently there is associated hyperextension with disruption of the disc spaces of the anterior longitudinal ligament, or of the anterior vertebral body. This injury, which involves all spinal columns, is unstable.

- Neurologic deficit depends upon a combination of the spinal cord injury at the time of the original fracture combined with the extent of persistent spinal cord compression.

- Conventional radiographs should be the initial imaging study. On lateral projections there may be anterior or posterior subluxation of the vertebra. On frontal projections a sagittal fracture through the vertebral body as well as possible fractures to lamina and facet joints can be seen. These fractures are more easily seen on CT scan.

- Similar to other spine fractures the full extent of osseous injury is not as well shown with routine radiographs as with CT scan.

- Soft tissue components of spinal injury are often better diagnosed using MRI. In particular, disc herniation may be appreciated with MRI and not with either non-contrast CT scan or conventional radiographs.

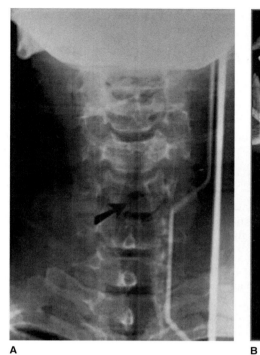

A

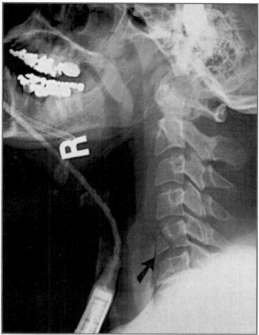

B

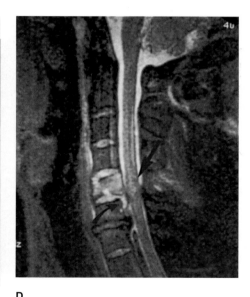

C   D

F I G U R E   3 0   **(A)** and **(B)** AP and lateral radiographs demonstrate the burst fracture of C5. The midline sagittal fracture can faintly be seen on the AP film *(arrows)*. **(C)** Axial CT section through the C5 vertebral body and C5-6 facet joints. Visible are the sagittal and coronal vertebral body fractures, bilateral laminar fractures, and bilateral widening of the C5-6 facet joints. **(D)** MRI of the cervical spine (T2-weighted fast spin echo with frequency-selective fat saturation) shows increased signal in C5 and in the C4-5 and C5-6 disc spaces. There is elevation of the posterior longitudinal ligament with protrusion of disc material into the spinal canal *(curved arrow)*. Increased signal is visible in the contused spinal cord *(arrow)*.

Suggested Reading

Pech P, Kilgore DP, Pojunas KW, Houghton VM. Cervical spine fractures: CT detection. *Radiology.* 1985;157:117–120.

Cervical Spine Injury: Unilateral Overriding Facet

KEY FACTS

- Unilateral facet override occurs from a combination of hyperflexion and rotation of the cervical spine.

- Patients may present with minimal neurologic deficit, root dysfunction or spinal cord dysfunction.

- Diagnosis is made using AP and lateral conventional radiographs. Commonly there will be a subluxation of less than 25% on the lateral projection. On the AP projection the spinous process above and below the level of injury will be out of alignment.

- Conventional radiographs are used to identify patients with injuries, while CT scanning is used to define the full extent of the fracture.

- With CT scan, diagnosis of unilateral facet override is made by noting the separation of articulating surfaces of the "jumped" facet joint if the patient has been reduced. In a non-reduced fracture, the flat, normally articulating surfaces of the facets face outward and the more rounded, non-articulating surfaces are opposed. Sagittal reformations are also helpful in demonstrating overriding facet positions.

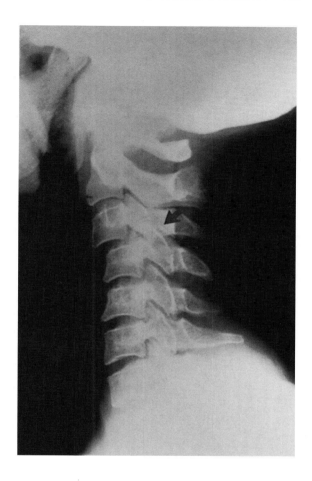

FIGURE 31

Lateral radiograph of the cervical spine
shows a unilateral overriding facet at C3-
4 *(arrow)*. Anterior subluxation of C3 on
C4 is approximately 25% *(arrow)*.

Suggested Reading

Gehweiler JA Jr., Osborne RL, Jr, Becker RF. *The Radiology of Vertebral Trauma*. Philadelphia: WB Saunders; 1980:239–252.

Cervical Spine Injury: Bilateral Overriding Facet

KEY FACTS

- This injury occurs with flexion/distraction forces to the cervical spine. There is disruption of ligaments and dislocation of the facet joints.

- Patients present with a range of neurologic dysfunction ranging from Frankel A (no detectable function below the level of injury) to Frankel E (normal neurologic examination).

- Similar to other spine trauma, the initial diagnostic study is a lateral radiograph of the cervical spine. As a first approximation, 50% or greater subluxation of one vertebral body anterior to the adjacent vertebra should suggest the presence of bilateral facet dislocation. There may be additional fractures present.

- Ligamentous injury is detected indirectly by noting widening of disc spaces and of the interspinous space between spinous processes.

- Cervical disc herniation is found in conjunction with bilateral facet dislocation in 2% to 30% of cases, depending upon the series.

- Initial management in spinal dislocation is reduction. This can precede more detailed imaging studies.

- CT is used to identify the extent of osseous injury. Fractures can be missed on routine radiographs. Use of CT as an initial screening study is currently under evaluation.

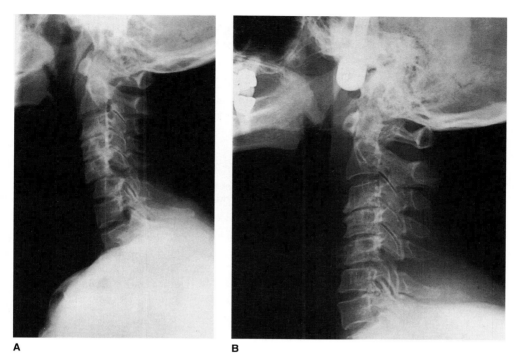

A   **B**

F I G U R E 3 2   **(A)** Lateral radiograph shows anterior subluxation of C5 on C6 with bilateral perched facets. **(B)** Lateral radiograph in traction following closed reduction. The C5/6 disc space is slightly wider posteriorly compared to the remainder of disc spaces. Facet joints and spinous process are separated.

Suggested Reading

Acheson MB, Livingston RR, Richardson ML, Stanao GK. High resolution CT scanning in evaluations of cervical spine trauma: A comparison with plain film examination. *AJR*. 1987;148:1179–1185.

Thoracic/Lumbar Spine Injury: Burst Fracture

KEY FACTS

- Burst fractures, the result of an axial load on the spinal column, are frequently found at the thoracolumbar junction. At a minimum there is disruption of the anterior and middle columns of the spine (minimal burst). When the injury is more severe, there may be disruption of all three columns.

- Anterior compression fractures, which also result from an axial load, involve only the anterior column.

- Mechanisms of injury include falls from heights, lesser falls in osteoporotic elderly patients, and motor vehicle accidents.

- Similar to other spine injuries, diagnosis is best made initially using conventional radiographs.

- Differentiation of burst fracture from anterior compression fracture requires demonstration of middle column injury. Although usually visible on conventional radiographs, when subtle this may be better appreciated with axial CT scans.

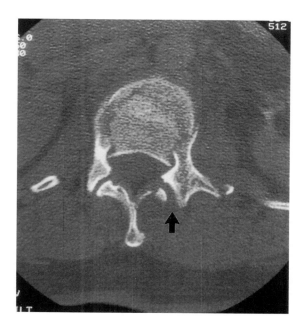

FIGURE 33

Axial CT scan through L1 shows fragmentation of the vertebral body, retropulsion of bone into the spinal canal with approximately 30% canal narrowing, and widening of the left T12-L1 facet joint *(arrow).*

Suggested Reading

Denis, F. The three-column spine and its significance in the classification of acute thora-columbar spinal injuries. *Spine.* 1983;8:817–831.

Thoracic/Lumbar Spine Injury: Flexion/Distraction Fracture

K E Y   F A C T S

- Sometimes called a "Chance-type" fracture, this injury has been associated with automobile lap belts and a rear seat position. The mechanism of injury is postulated to be hyperflexion. In a low-speed motor vehicle accident the lap belt, resting at the anterior abdominal wall, acts as the fulcrum of injury. In a high-speed motor vehicle accident, the fracture is postulated to be caused by the axial load associated with rapid deceleration.

- Greater than 50% of "Chance-type" fractures are associated with small bowel or colon injuries.

- The primary spinal injury is a horizontal fracture through the thoracolumbar spine, most commonly at L1-L3. There is minimal compression of the anterior column (vertebral body) combined with distraction of elements in the posterior column. This is an unstable injury.

- Similar to other spine trauma, initial imaging is best performed with conventional radiographs. CT is used to define the extent of the fracture and of spinal canal compromise.

- Because this fracture lies in an axial plane, it may be difficult to visualize with axial images. Diagnosis with CT may require sagittal and coronal reformations.

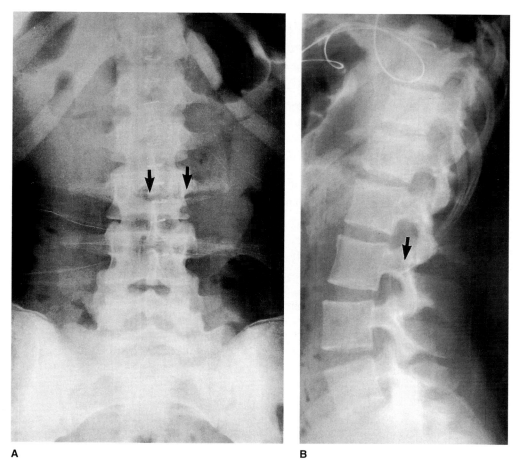

A   **B**

F I G U R E   3 4   **(A)** Radiograph of lumbar spine showing fracture line through the left transverse process and pedicle of L3 *(arrows)*. **(B)** Lateral radiograph has a minimal lucency through the pedicle and pars of L3 *(arrow)* with slight increase in height of the pedicle.

Suggested Reading

Anderson PA, Rivara FP, Maier RV, Drake C. The epidemiology of seatbelt-associated injuries. *J Trauma*. 1991;31:60–67.

Thoracic/Lumbar Spine Injury: Extension/ Distraction Fracture

KEY FACTS

- Extension-distraction injury occurs when hyperextension forces, often associated with rotation or shear, are applied to the spine. This is more common in the cervical than in the thoracic spine.

- Mechanisms of injury include falls backward or motor vehicle accidents.

- A patient with an ankylosed spine, irrespective of underlying etiology (such as degenerative disc disease or ankylosing spondylitis) is particularly subject to this injury.

- Typically there is greater disruption of the anterior column of the spine than of the posterior and middle columns. Facet joints and posterior arch may be fractured or dislocated. This injury is unstable.

- In the patient with ankylosed vertebral bodies, maintaining reduction of the fracture using external orthoses can be difficult. In these patients the spine on either side of the fracture acts biomechanically like two long lever arms.

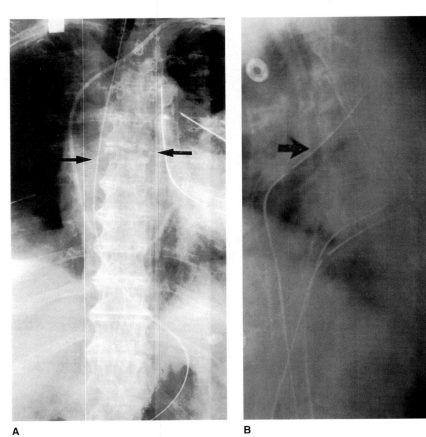

A   B

FIGURE 35   **(A)** and **(B)** AP and lateral radiographs show a fracture through C5 inferiorly *(arrows).* On the lateral projection there is a suggestion of anterior widening.

- Similar to other fractures that occur in an axial plane, diagnosis of flexion-distraction fracture is most easily made with lateral radiographs. If CT is used, the diagnosis is better appreciated on the sagittal and coronal reformatted images. With axial images, diagnosis can require observation of a missing normal osseous structure (the anterior portion of the vertebral body) rather than identification of a fracture line.

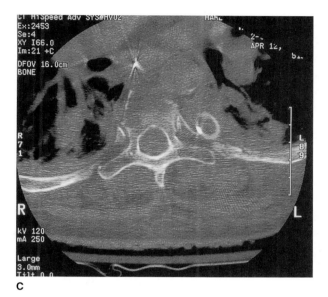

C

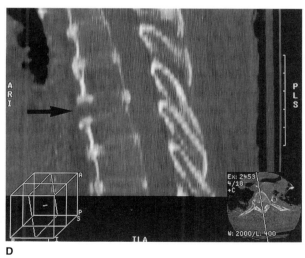

D

FIGURE 35 **(C)** Axial CT section through T5 is most remarkable for the absence of visible vertebral cortex anteriorly. **(D)** Sagittal reformatted CT scan better shows the widening anteriorly between C5 and C6 *(arrow)*.

Suggested Reading
Hendrix RW, Melany M, Miller F, Rogers LF. Fracture of the spine in patients with ankylosis due to diffuse skeletal hyperostosis: Clinical and imaging findings. *AJR*. 1994;162:899–904.

Radionuclide Detection of Cerebrospinal Fluid Leaks

KEY FACTS

- Radionuclide techniques are the most sensitive imaging tests for CSF leak detection.
- Scans integrate activity over time to detect and localize extra-neuraxial radionuclide activity that is indicative of leak.
- The radionuclide is instilled in the CSF usually via lumbar puncture.
- The preferred agent for CSF leak studies is In-111 DTPA because of its long half-life, but other radiotracers such as Tc-99m DTPA can be used as long as sterility and apyrogenicity is assured.
- Cotton pledgets may be placed in the nose, ears, or wounds, for example, and then measured in a well-counter for assay of radioactivity.
- If the leak may be in an unusual location, the use of single-photon tomography may aid in detection and localization.
- Abdominal images are obtained to evaluate for swallowed activity.
- The major morbidity expected from CSF leaks is infection.
- Once the leak is detected by the radionuclide study, other detailed imaging studies, such as CT myelography, may yield further localization.

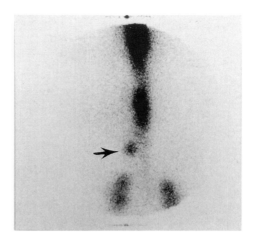

FIGURE 36

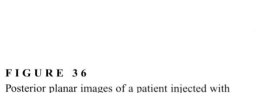

Posterior planar images of a patient injected with
In-111 DTPA via cervical puncture show
extravasation of radionuclide *(arrow)* to the bottom
left of the CSF column (above the left kidney).
Delayed image shows subtle accumulation of
radionuclide in the left hemithorax. The patient had
sustained a gunshot wound to the chest with
thoracic cord injury. Thoracostomy tube on left had
shown high rate of drainage.

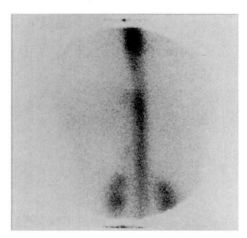

Suggested Reading

Lewis DH, Graham MM. Benefit of tomography in scintigraphic localization of cerebrospinal
fluid leak. *J Nucl Med*. 1991;32: 2149–2151.

TORSO

Scapulothoracic Dissociation

KEY FACTS

- Scapulothoracic dissociation is a rare but devastating closed forequarter amputation of the upper extremity in which severe traction or direct blow to the shoulder girdle results in near complete disruption of the forequarter to the torso. Brachial plexopathy, subclavian artery and venous injury are the rule.

- The vascular injuries associated with scapulothoracic dissociation are potentially limb or life threatening. Emergency subclavian arteriography is essential to assess the nature of arterial injuries to the limb in affected patients.

- Because most patients with this injury are involved in high-speed motor vehicle accidents, there is a high prevalence of other severe injuries.

- The important chest radiographic feature on a non-rotated film is laterally displaced scapula.
  - Check the scapulothoracic ratio (abnormal:normal, ≥ 1.40)

- Other clues to the diagnosis are:
  - Fracture of the clavicle with lateral displacement of several centimeters of the of the distal fragment
  - Acromioclavicular separation
  - Sternoclavicular fracture

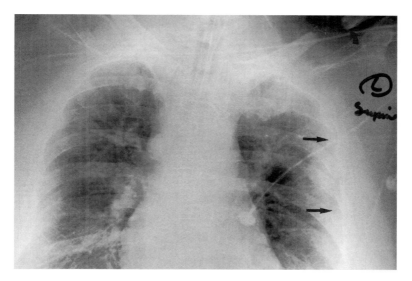

FIGURE 1   AP chest radiograph from a 49-year-old man involved in a high-speed motor vehicle accident shows multiple left rib fractures, a left clavicle fracture with associated lateral dislocation of the acromion *(curved arrow),* and lateral shift of the medial left scapular border *(arrows)* representing scapulothoracic dissociation. This is a very important finding to recognize as associated neurovascular injuries are potentially limb- or life-threatening. The scapulothoracic ratio compares the distances of the medial borders of the scapula to the midline. An abnormal ratio is ≥ 1.40. In this case, the ratio was 1.47.

Suggested Reading

Nagi ON, Dhillon MS. Traumatic scapulothoracic dissociation. A case report. *Arch Orthop Trauma Surg.* 1992;111:348–349.

Scapula Fracture

KEY FACTS

- Associated injuries are common with scapular fractures, including severe and life-threatening injuries in remote locations (such as the skull, abdomen, and pelvis), as well as major injuries to the adjacent chest and axilla.

- Rib fractures, pneumothorax, hemothorax, and lung contusion are frequent associates. Clavicle fractures are often found with glenoid injuries. Injuries to the brachial plexus and axillary vessels are infrequent, but when they do occur they have a poor prognosis.
  - 90% of patients with both scapular and rib fractures will also have a pneumothorax

- The severity of the other injuries often determines the management of a scapular fracture. Surgical repair may be delayed or ruled out in the face of life-threatening injuries elsewhere.

- Scapular fractures can cause apical-lateral pleural capping on chest radiographs, which should not be confused with the apical capping associated with mediastinal hematomas.

- Adequate radiographic evaluation of the scapula can be difficult, as much of the bone is often obscured by the chest on AP radiographs. AP and lateral views in the scapular plane (Grashey and "Y" views) are the minimum acceptable. Axillary views may be helpful in clarifying displacement and deformity.

- Adequate assessment of fracture morphology often requires CT. If surgical repair is planned, CT becomes an important part of the preoperative workup. Three-dimensional reconstructions are useful for surgical planning.

- The presence or absence of displacement, comminution, or articular involvement should always be determined. Intra-articular extension is often the deciding factor between surgical and conservative management.

- Displaced acromial, displaced glenoid, and severely displaced body and neck fractures will usually require surgical repair.

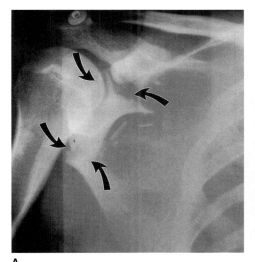

A

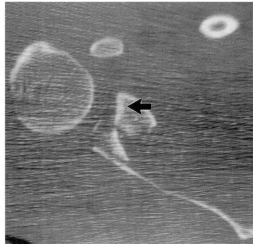

B

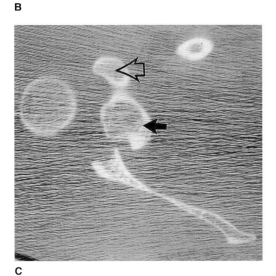

C

FIGURE 2

This patient fractured his scapula during a motor vehicle accident. The AP radiograph **(A)** shows the comminuted fracture of the scapula *(curved arrows)* extending through the glenoid fossa. CT scan through the central glenoid **(B)** shows the inferior portion of the glenoid *(arrow)* displaced medially. A second, more superior, CT scan slice **(C)** shows that the superior portion of the glenoid *(arrow),* with the coracoid process *(open arrow),* en face, because it is rotated 90° away from the humeral head. Surgery was necessary to restore the glenoid to a functional shape.

Suggested Reading

McGinnis M, Denton JR. Fractures of the scapula: A retrospective study of 40 fractured scapulae. *J Trauma.* 1989; 29:1488–1493.

Rib Fractures

KEY FACTS

- Usually follow blunt trauma to the chest, but also seen after vigorous coughing.

- Usually occur in the lower 10 ribs, laterally, away from the protection of the overlying chest wall musculature.

- First and second rib fractures occur after high kinetic energy absorption to the chest and can be associated with severe mediastinal and vascular injuries.

- Lower rib fractures are associated with increased risk of injury to the liver and spleen.

- Non-displaced rib fractures can be hard to visualize acutely on the chest radiograph, especially anterior fractures, often only revealing themselves as callous forms at the fracture site 10 to 14 days after injury. Rib cartilage fractures or separations are not radiographically evident.

- Specific radiographic examination of the ribs, with oblique positioning of the patient, is more accurate than the chest radiograph in detecting subtle rib fractures.

- Serious intrathoracic complications associated with rib fractures include pneumothorax, hemothorax, pulmonary contusion (see Figure 22), pulmonary laceration (see Figures 23 and 24), and secondarily, atelectasis, and pneumonia.

- Indirect radiographic findings, such as subpleural hematoma, increase the yield of a directed search for rib fracture.

Flail Chest

- Flail chest occurs when three or more ribs are each fractured in two places, also called segmental fractures.

- Flail chest serves as a marker of high kinetic energy absorption, but is not necessarily a marker for great vessel, tracheobronchial, or diaphragmatic injuries.

- Flail chest is highly associated with pulmonary contusion or laceration, pneumothorax, and hemothorax, especially with increasing number of rib fractures.

- Also associated with clavicular and scapular fractures.

- Most patients with flail chest require open reduction and internal fixation, and/or prolonged mechanical ventilation due to acute respiratory failure.

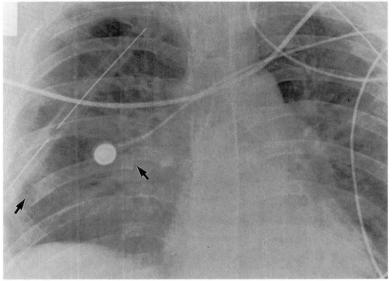

A

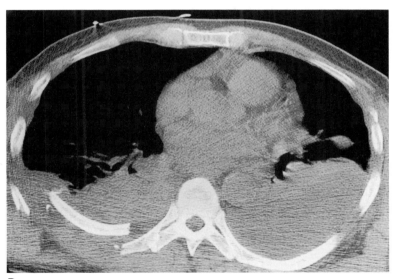

B

FIGURE 3 **(A)** AP chest radiograph from a 52-year-old man involved in a high-speed motor-vehicle accident shows multiple right ribs fractured in two places, posteriorly, with significant displacement *(arrows)*. **(B)** CT scan of the lower chest shows one of the right ribs fractured in two places, with significant inward displacement. Lung parenchymal opacities likely represent a combination of contusion and atelectasis.

Suggested Reading

Ciraulo DL, Elliott D, Mitchell KA, Rodriguez A. Flail chest as a marker for significant injuries. *J Am Coll Surg.* 1994; 178:466–470.

Sternoclavicular Dislocation

KEY FACTS

Anterior Sternoclavicular Dislocation

- Radiological examination has a limited value in diagnosing anterior sternoclavicular dislocations.

Posterior Sternoclavicular Dislocation

- Posterior sternoclavicular dislocation is a relatively rare form of trauma (<1% of all dislocations).

- Proximity of the clavicle to critical thoracic outlet structures can lead to severe or life-threatening complications, such as impingement on and possible injury to the trachea, esophageal injury, pneumothorax, laceration of underlying great vessels, and brachial plexus injury.

- Radiologic findings are similar for both anterior and posterior sternoclavicular dislocation and cannot be reliably distinguished.

- Radiologic findings can be subtle because there is only minimal displacement of the clavicle on the AP radiograph. On the *straight* supine AP chest radiograph look for:
  - Lateral displacement of the proximal end of the clavicle
  - Apparent asymmetry in clavicular head height

- Chest CT scanning is useful in quickly and accurately making the diagnosis.

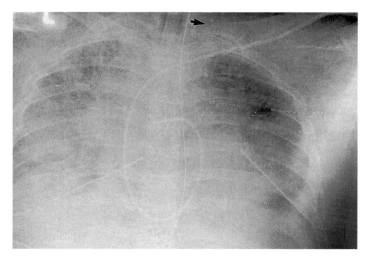

FIGURE 4   AP chest radiograph from a 35-year-old man involved in a motor-vehicle accident shows asymmetry of the clavicular head heights; the left clavicular head is displaced superiorly *(arrow)*.

Suggested Reading

Pearson MR, Leonard RB. Posterior sternoclavicular dislocation: A case report. *J Emerg Med.* 1994; 12:783–787.

Sternal and Manubrial Fractures

KEY FACTS

- The incidence of sternal fracture as a result of motor-vehicle collisions is about 3%, although the incidence may decrease with the advent of supplemental restraint devices (airbags).

- Pain and tenderness of the sternum are the most common patient complaints.

- Simple sternal fractures are usually benign and do not require special treatment or an expensive work-up.

- Depressed, segmental sternal fractures have an increased association with myocardial lacerations. Therefore, echocardiogram, to exclude pericardial effusion, is indicated (see acute traumatic hemopericardium).

- Manubrial fractures have a greater association with intrathoracic and upper mediastinal (especially great vessel) injuries.

- While there is an association with thoracic spine fractures and head trauma, sternal fractures are generally not associated with serious visceral chest injury; it is likely that the sternum absorbs a substantial part of the kinetic energy transferred in the injury, preventing greater underlying damage. This is not to say that serious myocardial, lung, airway, or diaphragm injuries never occur with sternal fracture.

- Fractures usually occur in the body of the sternum.

- Frontal chest radiographs usually do not show sternal fractures. Oblique or lateral chest radiographs are better at showing sternal fractures. Because sternal fractures can be impacted or overriding, they can appear on oblique views as linear bands of increased density (not lucent).

- Chest CT scanning is not generally indicated in most patients, but can clearly show sternal fractures, as well as associated mediastinal injuries, such as presence of hematoma or hemopericardium.

- The outcome of patients with an isolated sternal fracture and a normal ECG is very good (see Myocardial Contusion).

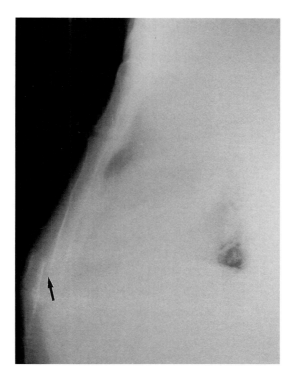

FIGURE 5

Lateral chest radiograph from a 69-year-old man involved in a motor-vehicle accident, complaining of chest wall pain and tenderness, shows a depressed, complete fracture of the distal sternum *(arrow)*. This man had no other associated mediastinal injuries.

Suggested Reading

Hills MW, Delprado AM, Deane SA. Sternal fractures: Associated injuries and management. *J Trauma.* 1993;35:55–60.

Airway Rupture/Laceration

KEY FACTS

Cervical Trachea

- These injuries usually occur secondary to a direct blow, most frequently a steering wheel.
- There is a range of injury severity from membranous rupture, to cartilage ring fracture, to cricothyroid dislocation.
- Direct laryngoscopy and open exploration are indicated for severe injuries.
- CT scanning is a useful modality for lesser injuries; look for abnormal air collections, cartilage fractures, and arytenoid dislocations.

Intrathoracic Trachea

- Airway disruptions can be due to both blunt and penetrating injuries, though are infrequent after blunt chest trauma, with an incidence of about 1%.
- The clinical picture is not uniform, hence the correct diagnosis can be delayed.
- Patients typically exhibit cough, significant soft tissue emphysema, pneumomediastinum, pneumothorax, hemoptysis, increasing respiratory distress, and hypoxia within a few hours of the injury.
- The most common sites of injury are the main bronchi (right > left), 75% occur within 2 cm of the tracheal carina.
- Tracheobronchial rupture from blunt trauma is usually single and transverse, but a minority may have longitudinal or complex tears.
- Associated injuries include first or second rib fractures, rupture of the great vessels, and traumatic false aneurysm of a pulmonary artery.
- While often suspected radiographically, the diagnosis is usually confirmed endo/bronchoscopically.
- Chest radiographs show:
    - Extensive soft tissue emphysema
    - Pneumomediastinum
    - Pneumothorax that fails to re-expand with chest tube drainage
- With tracheal lacerations, mediastinal air collections will predominate. >2 cm from the tracheal carina, recalcitrant pneumothorax will predominate. Within 2 cm of the tracheal carina, heterotopic air collections will be mixed.
- A rare, but pathognomonic chest radiographic finding is the so-called fallen lung sign on the upright chest radiograph; after a complete laceration of a main bronchus, the lung collapses, or falls, down into the dependent pleural space.

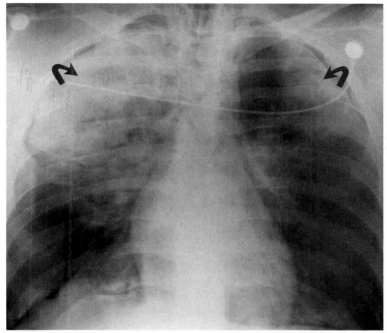

A

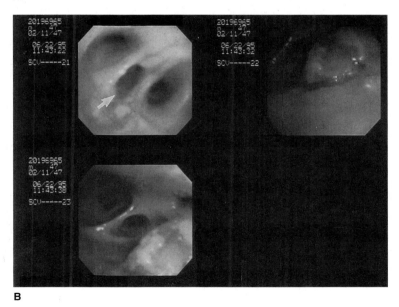

B

FIGURE 6   **(A)** Initial AP chest radiograph from a 20-year-old man who jumped off a 50-meter bridge shows multiple features of barotrauma: pneumomediastinum, bilateral pneumothoraces, as well as bilateral apical parenchymal opacities that likely represent pulmonary contusion *(curved arrows).* Because of the mechanism of injury (severe deceleration), clinical suspicion, and persistent pneumothoraces and pneumomediastinum, bronchoscopy was performed and showed a laceration of the left upper lobe bronchus. **(B)** Bronchoscopic view of a lacerated airway, from a similar patient, shows a relatively distal bronchial tear between the right middle lobe and right lower lobe segmental bronchus *(arrow).*

Suggested Reading

Symbas PN, Justicz AG, Ricketts RR. Rupture of the airways from blunt trauma: Treatment of complex injuries. *Ann Thorac Surg.* 1992;54:177–183.

Esophageal Rupture/Laceration

KEY FACTS

- Esophageal rupture can occur either due to blunt (very rare) or penetrating injuries, as well as, be a complication of instrumentation and vigorous emesis.

- Blunt injuries are usually seen in the phrenic ampulla and cervical esophagus, while penetrating injuries can occur anywhere, depending on the location of the entrance wound.

- Esophageal rupture can also be seen in blast injuries.

- Penetrating injuries that traverse the mediastinum require assessment of the great vessels (angiography), trachea (bronchoscopy), and esophagus (endoscopy and/or esophagography). Classically, each misses one third of injuries, but not the same third.

- In penetrating injuries of the supraclavicular esophagus, the trachea is injured in half of cases (and vice versa).

- Delay in diagnosing esophageal rupture doubles patient mortality every 6 hours; >85% mortality if the delay is >24 hours.

- Chest radiographs are non-specific, and usually show a wide mediastinum and left pleural effusion or hydropneumothorax. Pneumomediastinum is another common, non-specific finding. Occasionally, one can see the "V-sign of Naclerio," where pneumomediastinum extends to and reflects the parietal pleura off the left hemidiaphragm yielding a lucent "V" (see Figure 30).

- Pleural effusion will often show a low pH and high amylase levels.

- Mediastinitis and abscess formation can result from an esophageal laceration.

- For esophagographic diagnosis of esophageal rupture, use non-ionic contrast (300 mg I/ml) in the LAO position. If this is normal, follow with thin barium solution in the LAO and RAO positions (see page 42).

Suggested Reading
Bjerke HS. Penetrating and blunt injuries of the esophagus. *Chest Surg Clin N Am.* 1994;4: 811–818.

Esophageal Intubation with Gastric Perforation

KEY FACTS

- Unrecognized esophageal malposition is an uncommon (≤1%) but potentially catastrophic complication of attempted endotracheal intubation.

- Esophageal intubation is diagnosed on chest radiographs by showing:
  - Projection of any part of the endotracheal tube outside of the tracheo-bronchial air column
  - An enlarged tracheal balloon cuff (transverse diameter >2.8 cm)
  - New extrapulmonary gas collections (marked gastric dilation, pneumoperitoneum, pneumomediastinum)
  - Distal prolapse of the tracheal balloon (distal margin <1.2 cm proximal to endotracheal tube tip)

- Chest radiographs should be obtained routinely to verify correct endotracheal tube position.

- Gastric rupture and pneumoperitoneum following esophageal intubation and ventilation is rare, usually occurring during cardiopulmonary resuscitation.

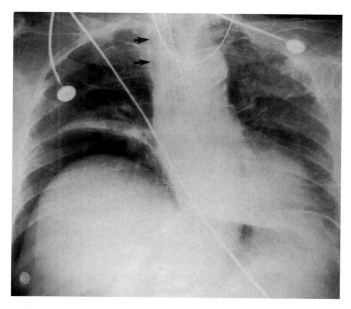

FIGURE 7   AP chest radiograph from an 80-year-old-woman after accidental esophageal intubation shows a large pneumoperitoneum resulting from gastric rupture. Note the endotracheal balloon cuff projecting beyond the tracheal air column *(arrows)*. (From Song JK, et al. Gastric perforation: a complication of inadvertent esophageal intubation. *AJR* 1995;164:1386, with permission.)

Suggested Reading

Brunel W, Coleman DL, Schwartz DE, Peper E, Cohen NH. Assessment of routine chest roentgenograms and the physical examination to confirm endotracheal tube position. *Chest.* 1989;96:1043–1045.

Traumatic Aortic Injury: Chest Radiography

KEY FACTS

- Blunt traumatic injury to the thoracic aorta accounts for 10 to 20% of fatalities in high-speed deceleration accidents; 80 to 90% of these victims die at the accident scene.

- Of the 10% to 20% of patients that reach the hospital; 30% die within 6 hours, 40% to 50% die within 24 hours and 90% die within 4 months if the aortic injury is not discovered and repaired.

- Traumatic thoracic aortic injuries occur most commonly at the aortic isthmus (80%–85%), followed by the ascending aortic arch (5%–9%), great vessels (4%–10%), and diaphragmatic hiatus (1%–3%).

- Chronic posttraumatic thoracic aortic pseudoaneurysm develops in 2% to 5% of patients with this injury. Only rarely do these patients live a normal life-span.

- There are many chest radiographic signs used to detect mediastinal hematoma; no individual sign is specific for acute traumatic aortic injury (ATAI). The mechanism of injury and clinical suspicion are still very important factors. The basic premise is that 99% of ATAI are associated with mediastinal hematoma. Well-recognized chest radiographic signs of mediastinal hematoma, and thus indirectly ATAI, include:
  - Superior mediastinal widening (>8 cm) at the aortic knob
  - Abnormal aortic contour
  - Aortopulmonary window opacification
  - Deviation of trachea, nasogastric tube, or endotracheal tube to the right
  - Abnormal left paraspinal "stripe"
  - Thickened right paratracheal "stripe"
  - Depression of left main bronchus
  - Left hemothorax

- Mediastinal widening on the chest radiograph is the most sensitive diagnostic sign for traumatic aortic injury (92%), however, by itself, it is not that useful, with a specificity of only 10%. Mediastinal widening can be the result of magnification and distortion of the mediastinal contour inherent in the portable supine chest radiograph. It can also be due to atherosclerosis, mediastinal lipomatosis, pulmonary atelectasis, or pleural effusions abutting the mediastinum or mediastinal lymph adenopathy.

- The negative predictive value of a normal chest radiograph is 98%, in other words, it "virtually" excludes the presence of aortic injury.

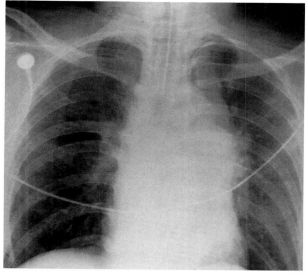

A

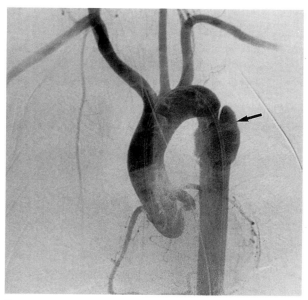

B

F I G U R E 8   **(A)** AP chest radiograph from a 21-year-old-man involved in a high-speed motor-vehicle accident shows superior mediastinal widening and loss of the normally sharp aortic contour. These findings, as well as the mechanism of injury indicated aortography. **(B)** Left anterior oblique aortic angiogram shows a typical aortic laceration at the aortic isthmus *(arrow).*

Suggested Reading

Woodring JH. The normal mediastinum in blunt traumatic rupture of the thoracic aorta and brachiocephalic arteries. *J Emerg Med.* 1990;8:467–476.

Acute Traumatic Aortic Injury: Angiographic Pitfalls

KEY FACTS

- The angiographic diagnosis of ATAI rests on the demonstration of an intimal irregularity or intraluminal filling defect that represents an intimal flap, or on the appearance of contrast material outside the projected lumen of the aorta representing a pseudoaneurysm. The specificity of aortography for ATAI is 99% to 100%. Although cases of false negative aortograms have been reported, the sensitivity approaches 100%.

- Atypical or equivocal angiographic findings for ATAI are encountered in 1% to 5% of the cases, and may lead to unnecessary thoracotomy or delayed surgical management. These false results are due to:
  - Anatomical variants
  - Atheromatous plaques
  - Syphilitic aortic aneurysm
  - Artifacts from physiologic streaming/mixing of contrast media, motion, and digital subtraction

- Important anatomic variants include ductus diverticulum (incidence 9%–33%), aortic spindle (incidence 16%) and a prominent infundibulum of the bronchial-intercostal trunk. These can be easily confused with a pseudoaneurysm. Angiographically, a ductus diverticulum is smooth, has obtuse margins with the aortic wall and there is no delay in washout of the contrast. Rarely, a ductus diverticulum can fold back against the aorta creating the appearance of an intimal flap. The aortic spindle is a smooth fusiform dilatation distal to the isthmus. Discrimination of a prominent infundibulum of the bronchial artery from a traumatic pseudoaneurysm requires demonstration of an arterial branch arising from it.

- Atherosclerotic intimal elevation can mimic an intimal flap. The surface depression of an ulcerated atheromatous plaque and the extraluminal contrast collection within a penetrating atherosclerotic ulcer of the thoracic aorta can mimic a pseudoaneurysm. Angiographically there is a focal outpouching with smooth intrinsic impression of the aortic wall representing the elevated intima by atheroma. Contrast enhanced CT is helpful if it demonstrates ulcerated atheromatous plaque, but no focal periaortic hematoma, or a penetrating ulcer with heaped-up margins and inward displacement of intimal calcifications and no focal periaortic hematoma.

- Complementary imaging by intravascular ultrasound may be helpful in equivocal cases.

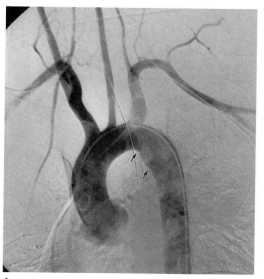
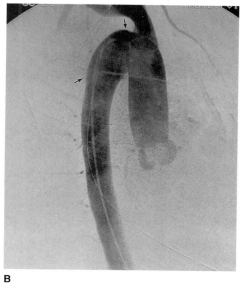

A   **B**

F I G U R E   9   Two patients with **(A)** ductus diverticulum and **(B)** aortic spindle, respectively. On aortography, both are smooth, focal outpouchings and their margins form obtuse angles *(arrows)* with the aortic wall. Also there is no delay in washout of the contrast.

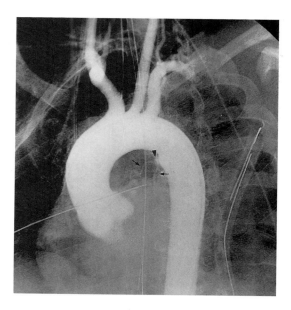

F I G U R E   1 0

Prominent infundibulum *(arrowhead)* of the bronchial trunk superimposed on a small ductus diverticulum. Note the bronchial arteries *(arrows)* emanating from the infundibulum.

Acute Traumatic Aortic Injury: Angiographic Pitfalls *(Continued)*

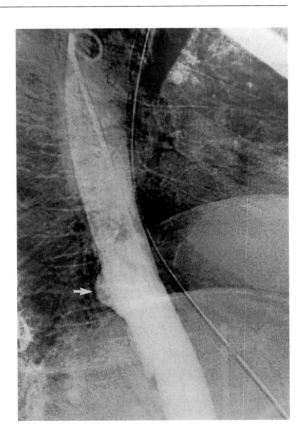

FIGURE 11
Penetrating ulcer of the descending thoracic aorta.

Suggested Reading

Morse SS, Glickman MG, Greenwood LH, et al. Traumatic aortic rupture: False-positive aortographic diagnosis due to atypical ductus diverticulum. *AJR.* 1988;150(4):793–796.

Traumatic Aortic Injury: Computed Tomography

KEY FACTS

- The role of CT scanning in evaluating patients with suspected ATAI is controversial.

- Most authors agree that CT scanning is superior to chest radiography in depicting mediastinal hematoma. Mirvis et al. found that when mediastinal hematoma was used as an indirect CT sign of ATAI, the sensitivity is 100%, specificity is 87%, positive predictive value is 21% and a negative predictive value based upon clinical outcome is 100%. The mediastinal hematoma of ATAI is either contiguous with the aorta or periaortic.

- Direct CT scan signs of ATAI are pseudoaneurysm, intraluminal filling defect/intimal flap, irregular aortic contour, pseudocoarctation and dissection. Using direct CT scan signs of ATAI, CT scanning has a sensitivity of 90% to 100% and a specificity of 81.7% to 98.6%. Visualizing injuries to the proximal ascending aorta and brachiocephalic vessels is problematic.

- CT scans are obtained sequentially from the base of the neck to the diaphragm. By conventional CT scan methods, imaging is sequentially obtained at 5 to 10 mm thickness slices. By helical CT scan methods, the parameters are usually 7 mm slice-thickness and table speed of 7 mm/sec (pitch = 1) with retrospective reconstruction every 3.5 mm (50% overlap). Intravenous iodinated contrast is administered with a power injector at a rate of 1.5 to 2.0 cc/sec for a total volume of 100 to 150 ml, with a 20 to 30-second scan delay.

- Equivocal, indeterminate, and false results of CT scanning can be attributable to suboptimal exam, artifacts (motion, aortic pulsation, linear streak), volume averaging, normal variants (ductus diverticulum, aortic spindle, prominent infundibulum of bronchial artery), prominent para-aortic mediastinal vessels, prominent atheromatous plaque, para-aortic atelectasis or effusion, and thymic tissue. To minimize CT scan artifacts, ECG leads must be appropriately positioned, patient removed from the backboard if possible, the patient's arms raised over his head and images obtained during suspended respiration.

- If there is any abnormality on the CT scan that is not 100% directly diagnostic of ATAI, transcatheter aortography is necessary.

Traumatic Aortic Injury: Computed Tomography
(Continued)

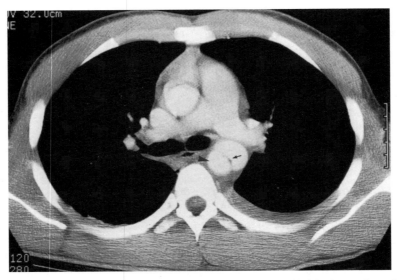

F I G U R E   1 2   CT scan of a typical traumatic aortic tear *(arrow)* and false lumen *(arrowhead)* involving the proximal descending thoracic aorta in a hemodynamically stable 23-year-old man involved in a motor-vehicle accident. Note the para-aortic hematoma and left hemothorax.

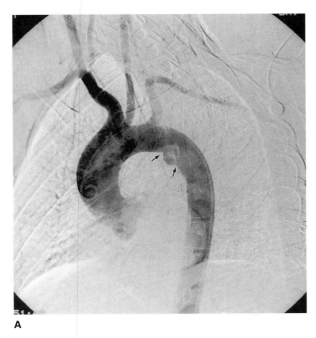

A

F I G U R E   1 3   Aortography in a hemodynamically stable 42-year-old man struck by a falling tree. **(A)** shows a focal, smooth outpouching of the thoracic aorta in the expected location of the ductus diverticulum. There is no delay in washout of contrast, however, its margins with the aortic wall are acute *(arrows)* rather than obtuse.

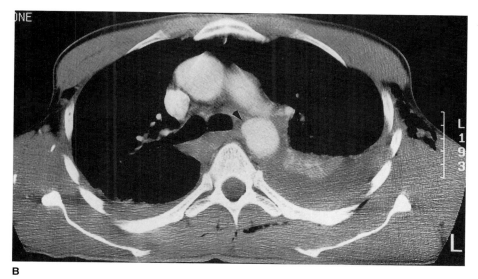

FIGURE 13 **(B)** CT scan shows para-aortic hematoma *(arrowhead)* and bilateral pleural effusions. **(C)** Intravascular ultrasonography shows the tear *(arrows)* and false lumen *(arrowhead).*

Suggested Reading

Mirvis SE, Shanmuganathan K, Miller BH, White CS, Turney SZ. Traumatic aortic injury: Diagnosis with contrast-enhanced thoracic CT—Five-year experience at a major trauma center. *Radiology.* 1996;200(2):413–422.

Traumatic Aortic Injury: Transesophageal Echocardiography

KEY FACTS

- Direct signs of aortic injury on transesophageal echocardiography (TEE) is demonstration of an intimal flap, a false lumen (pseudoaneurysm), an aortic wall disruption (complete transection) or an aortic wall hematoma (subintimal, medial, or subadventitial).

- Studies on TEE depiction of ATAI have yielded a sensitivity of 57% to 100% and specificity of 84% to 100%.

- TEE is portable and can be performed at the patient's bedside. TEE requires a skilled and experienced operator for proper manipulation of the probe and for proper acquisition and interpretation of the images. Because the descending aorta is scanned in close proximity to the esophagus, the potential exists for near-field artifacts caused by excessive gain and reverberation.

- The ascending aorta around the trachea and left mainstem bronchus, a 3 to 5 cm portion, is not well seen and is called the "blind spot." Artifacts, atheromatous plaque, and extensive atherosclerotic disease can produce false-positive or equivocal results. TEE performed with a biplane/multiplane probe with Doppler interrogation and color flow mapping helps reduce artifact errors and minimizes the "blind spot." Visualization of the brachiocephalic vessels is another major limitation of TEE.

- TEE should not be attempted in patients who are combative, have unstable neck or spine injuries, have acute or chronic esophageal disease, have severe maxillofacial trauma, or have suspected injury to the brachiocephalic vessels.

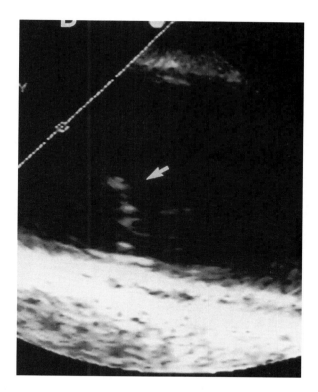

FIGURE 14

Simple traumatic initmal tear *(arrow)* of the proximal descending aorta.

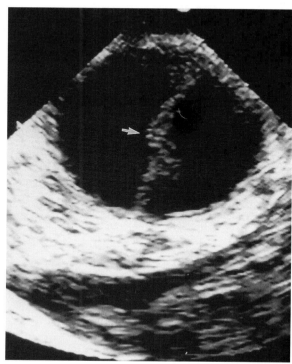

FIGURE 15

Traumatic aortic transection. Note tear *(arrow)* with a false lumen at the isthmus.

Suggested Reading

Minard G, Schurr MJ, Croce MA, et al. A prospective analysis of transesophageal echocardiography in the diagnosis of traumatic disruption of the aorta. *J of Trauma.* 1996;40(2): 225–230.

Injury to Brachiocephalic Vessels

KEY FACTS

- Injury to the innominate or subclavian artery is an uncommon problem that can occur secondary to both blunt (see also scapulothoracic dissociation and sternal/manubrial fractures) and penetrating injuries.

- In blunt chest trauma, isolated brachiocephalic vessel injury is rare; these injuries are more commonly associated with aortic injuries and, unlike penetrating injuries, usually occur at their origin.

- In blunt trauma, brachiocephalic vessel injury (not aorta) is associated with manubrial fractures (10%) and posterior left sternoclavicular dislocations (10%), and scapulothoracic dissociation.

- Patients with penetrating injury are more unstable at presentation than patients with blunt injuries and the mortality is much higher.

- General indications for angiography with penetrating injuries:
  - Stable zone I (torso or neck) injuries
  - Angiography rather than surgical exploration if the location of injury requires two field exposure (e.g., neck and chest)

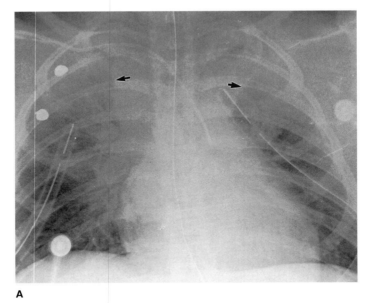

A

FIGURE 16   (A) AP chest radiograph from an 13-year-old-boy who sustained several gunshot wounds to the chest shows mediastinal widening, with the mediastinal contours, convex laterally *(arrows).* Incidental note is made of a central venous catheter inadvertently placed in the aorta.

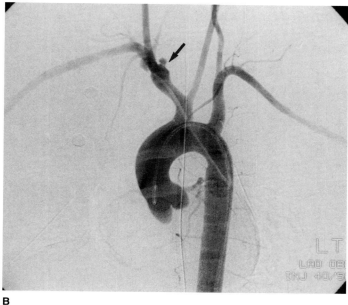

FIGURE 16 **(B)** Left anterior oblique aortic angiogram shows a post-traumatic subclavian artery pseudoaneurysm, with no active leaking of contrast *(arrow)*.

Suggested Reading
Hoff SJ, Reilly MK, Merrill WH, Stewart J, Frist WH, Morris JAJ. Analysis of blunt and penetrating injury of the innominate and subclavian arteries. *Am Surg.* 1994;60:151–154.

Myocardial Contusion

KEY FACTS

- Myocardial contusions result from rapid deceleration or application of great force to the anterior chest, as occurs in motor-vehicle accidents with the anterior chest striking the steering wheel.

- Myocardial contusions are considered to be an intramural hematoma in the myocardial wall.

- Sternal fractures are commonly, but not exclusively, associated with myocardial contusion.

- Myocardial contusions remain difficult to diagnose, however, diagnosis is vital in unstable patients, as well as in hemodynamically stable patients, despite its low morbidity.

- Diagnosis is usually made by one or a combination of four diagnostic procedures: electrocardiography, echocardiography, creatine phosphokinase MB isoenzyme fractions, or thallium-201 scintigraphy; though some authors advocate using just electrocardiography and careful physical examination because serum myocardial enzymes and radionuclide studies are nonspecific and are not predictive of cardiac complications.

- Chest radiographs are of little value in diagnosis of myocardial contusion, but are useful in finding associated injuries as markers of injury severity such as flail chest, sternal fracture, and pulmonary contusion.

- Echocardiography is useful in the management of myocardial decompensation, but not as a primary screening tool in blunt cardiac injury. Findings include:
  - Pericardial effusion
  - Regional wall motion abnormalities
  - Pneumopericardium
  - Intramyocardial hematoma in the free wall of the right ventricle
  - Decreased ejection fraction

- The incidence of clinically significant supraventricular or ventricular dysrhythmias or other cardiac complications, such as congestive failure, resulting from myocardial contusion is overestimated.

- Coronary artery laceration and thrombosis is a very rare complication.

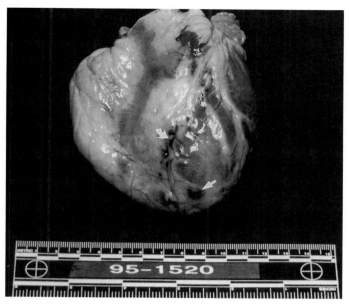

FIGURE 17   Gross autopsy specimen of the heart of a 16-year-old child involved in a fatal high-speed motor-vehicle accident shows myocardial contusions over the anterior surface of the heart *(arrow)*. Incidental note was made of a rare complication of severe blunt injury to the heart, laceration of the left anterior descending coronary artery *(curved arrow)*. (Case courtesy of Richard C. Harruff. Seattle, WA).

Suggested Reading

McLean RF, Devitt JH, McLellan BA, Dubbin J, Ehrlich LE, Dirkson D. Significance of myocardial contusion following blunt chest trauma. *J Trauma.* 1992;33:240–243.

Cardiac Perforation and Rupture

KEY FACTS

- Cardiac rupture can occur from either penetrating injuries to the chest, such as stab or gunshot wounds, or from severe blunt trauma to the chest, usually anteriorly.

- Blunt traumatic cardiac rupture is associated with a high rate of mortality and most frequently results from motor-vehicle accidents, crush injuries and falls.

- The mean Injury Severity and Trauma Scores are usually very high.

- Severe blunt trauma can lead to right atrial rupture (most common), followed by right ventricular rupture, left atrial rupture and, least commonly, left ventricular rupture.

- The overall mortality rate is >80% for single atrial chamber rupture, and 100% with multi-chamber rupture.

- Survivors usually have a small rupture with a slow, contained leak.

- Diagnosis is usually made by emergent thoracotomy. Imaging plays almost no role; chest CT scanning rarely makes the diagnosis, usually serendipitously.

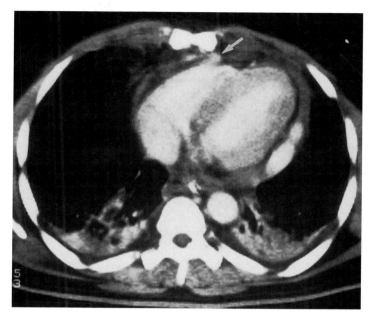

FIGURE 18   CT scan of the chest from a patient with severe chest trauma shows a small outpouching of blood from the anterior wall of the right ventricle *(arrow)* and an associated small pericardial effusion as evidence of right ventricular rupture, confirmed surgically. (Case courtesy of Stuart E. Mirvis, University of Maryland).

Suggested Reading

Brathwaite CE, Rodriguez A, Turney SZ, Dunham CM, Cowley R. Blunt traumatic cardiac rupture. A 5-year experience. *Ann Surg.* 1990;212:701–704.

Acute Traumatic Hemopericardium

KEY FACTS

- Blunt chest trauma can result in cardiac concussion, contusion, and rupture; cardiac valvular dysfunction; aortic laceration; and hemopericardium that may be complicated by cardiac tamponade.

- Acute traumatic hemopericardium usually results from pericardial or myocardial contusion, or aortic root rupture.

- In the absence of cardiac tamponade, arrhythmias, or congestive heart failure, most cases of isolated traumatic hemopericardium resolve uneventfully.

- Constrictive pericarditis can be a serious, late complication that typically occurs weeks or months after the event, possibly secondary to the post-cardiac injury syndrome.

- The diagnosis is usually made by clinical suspicion, and by chest CT scanning or echocardiography.

- The chest radiograph is limited in diagnosing hemopericardium; look for enlarged, globular cardiac contour, though this is a non-specific and insensitive finding. Secondary findings of left heart congestive failure are also non-specific.

- The chest radiograph is more useful after the diagnosis is made by detecting complications such as congestive failure, and by detecting other associated injuries as markers of injury severity such as flail chest, sternal fracture, and pulmonary contusion.

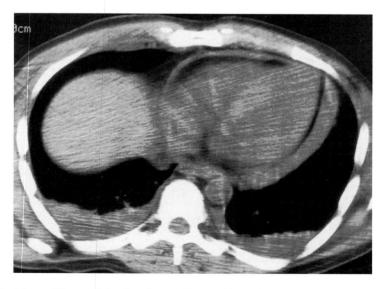

FIGURE 19   CT scan of the chest from a 40-year-old-man involved in a head-on motor-vehicle accident shows a fluid collection within the pericardial space. The CT attenuation of the pericardial fluid is similar to the blood within the left ventricle (30 Hounsfield Units). (From Stern EJ, Frank MS. Acute traumatic hemopericardium. *AJR* 1994;162:1305–1306, with permission.)

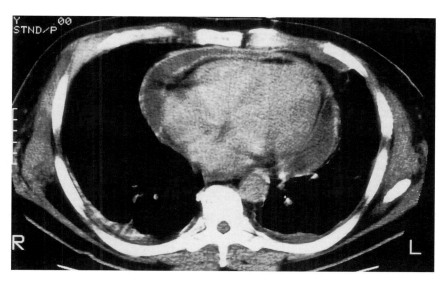

F I G U R E   2 0   Contrast-enhanced CT scan from 56-year-old-man involved in a motor-vehicle accident 4 weeks prior to presentation, now with clinical signs and symptoms of constrictive pericarditis, shows a fluid collection within the pericardial space. The pericardium is thickened and enhanced, consistent with pericarditis. (From Stern EJ, Frank MS. Acute traumatic hemopericardium. *AJR* 1994;162:1305–1306, with permission.)

Suggested Reading

Harman P, Trinkle J. Injuries to the heart. In *Trauma*. 2nd ed.. Norwalk, CT: Appleton and Lange; 1991:373–391.

Hemidiaphragm Injury

KEY FACTS

- Hemidiaphragm rupture can occur following both blunt and penetrating mechanisms of injury. In blunt injury, high intra-abdominal pressures are speculated as the usual mechanism of hemidiaphragm rupture, although penetrating rib fractures can also lacerate the hemidiaphragm.

- Incidence of right-sided versus left-sided hemidiaphragm rupture, after blunt abdominal trauma is controversial. The classic teaching is that 90% of ruptures are left-sided, however, the true incidence may be more equal, the liver just preventing clinical manifestations.

- 90% of clinically significant hemidiaphragm ruptures are overlooked initially and 90% of strangulated diaphragmatic hernias are of traumatic etiology.

- Hemidiaphragm rupture can occur in the acute trauma setting or be delayed by days, weeks, or even years.

- Hemidiaphragm rupture is associated with other significant intra-abdominal injuries in most cases.

- Small lacerations of the hemidiaphragm are hard to detect; the chest radiograph can be normal.

- With a large hemidiaphragm rupture, chest radiographs are never normal. Radiographic findings of left hemidiaphragm rupture include:
  - Loops of bowel, usually stomach and colon, within the thorax
  - Nasogastric tube showing the position of the stomach within the thorax
  - Left pleural effusion
  - Ill-defined soft-tissue mass obscuring the left hemidiaphragm
  - Left basilar lung atelectasis

  Radiographic findings of right hemidiaphragm rupture include:
  - Apparent elevation of the hemidiaphragm
  - Pleural effusion
  - Rarely, loops of bowel or the entire liver within the thorax (must be a very large laceration)

- CT and MRI scans can be used as adjunctive diagnostic tests in difficult cases, especially using coronal imaging planes.

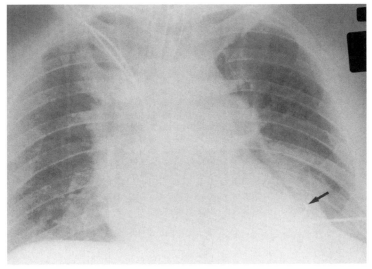

A

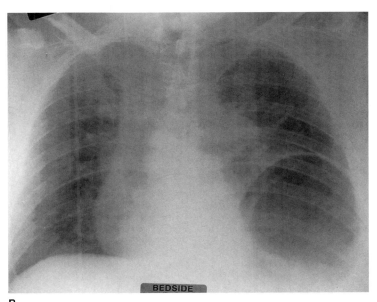

B

FIGURE 21 **(A)** Initial AP chest radiograph from a 37-year-old-man involved in a motor-vehicle accident shows obscuration of the left hemidiaphragm, with the nasogastric tube extending slightly above the expected position of the hemidiaphragm contour *(arrow).* **(B)** AP chest radiograph obtained 12 hours later shows marked distention of the stomach apparently within the thorax. Hemidiaphragm rupture was strongly suspected, and confirmed surgically.

Suggested Reading

Gelman R, Mirvis SE, Gens D. Diaphragmatic rupture due to blunt trauma: Sensitivity of plain chest radiographs. *AJR.* 1991;156:51–57.

Pulmonary Contusion

KEY FACTS

- The most common traumatic lung injury is a bruise or pulmonary contusion.

- Unlike bruising one's shin, it takes a significant amount of energy absorption to bruise the lung; a pulmonary contusion is a marker of injury severity.

- Pulmonary contusion occurs in both blunt and penetrating injuries, with or without rib fractures, and from blast injuries. They are also caused by shearing forces (variable rates of deceleration that compress and stretch the lung).

- Contusions can cause dyspnea, tachycardia, and hypoxia. Hemoptysis is uncommon.

- Mortality rates of up to 31% have been reported in patients with massive pulmonary contusions, and they play a major role in up to one quarter of motor-vehicle accident fatalities.

- Pulmonary contusions caused by stab or gunshot wounds are usually small and clinically inconsequential, the exception being shotgun wounds that can have a pronounced blast effect (see Figure 28).

- Pulmonary contusions are seen radiographically within 6 hours of injury in up to 85% of patients, and in 100% of patients within 12 to 24 hours, and show:
    - Patchy, nonsegmental, ill-defined parenchymal opacity, usually with no anatomic boundary
    - Opacities are peripheral and under the point of injury
    - Opacities can be scattered, or coup or contracoup

- Pulmonary contusions start clearing in 2 to 3 days—it is a dynamic process that usually resolves within 4 to 5 days (range 1 to 10 days). CT scanning is generally not indicated.

- When new lung parenchymal opacities appear >24 hours after injury, strongly consider other etiologies such as aspiration or superimposed infection.

- Pulmonary contusions can be an independent injury that resolves to leave the chest radiograph normal, however, they can initially mask more serious underlying injuries that only appear as the contusions resolve (e.g., lacerations with resulting pneumatoceles or hematomas).

- Conversely, pulmonary contusions can be masked by other injuries (e.g., pneumothorax, hemothorax, etc.).

- Basilar pulmonary contusions, especially with associated rib fractures, should alert the radiologist to associated *intra-abdominal* injuries.

Pulmonary Contusion (Continued)

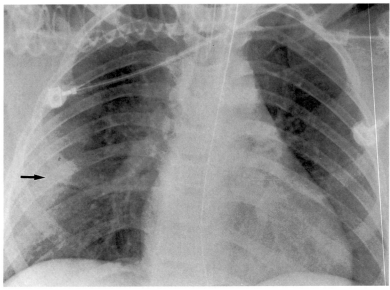

A

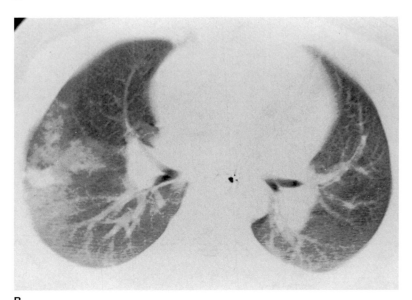

B

FIGURE 22   (A) AP chest radiograph from a 12-year-old-boy, involved in a motor-vehicle accident, shows an ill-defined peripheral opacity in the right lung *(arrow)* consistent with a pulmonary contusion. (B) CT scan of the chest performed the same day confirms the ill-defined, non-anatomic, peripheral nature of the contusions, with no evidence of underlying pulmonary laceration, or other intrathoracic injury.

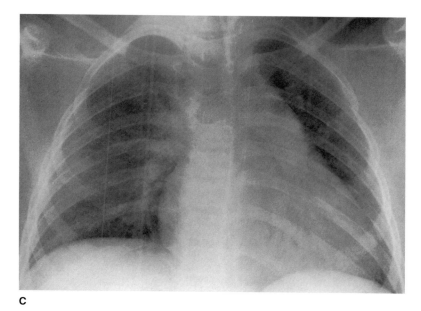

C

FIGURE 22 (C) AP chest radiograph obtained 4 days after injury shows complete resolution of the pulmonary contusion.

Suggested Reading

Groskin, S. *Radiological, Clinical and Biomechanical Aspects of Chest Trauma.* Berlin: Springer Verlag; 1991.

Pulmonary Laceration

KEY FACTS

- The term pulmonary laceration implies frank disruption of lung tissue causing a localized internal leak of air (pneumatocele) and blood (hematoma) in variable quantities.

- A pulmonary laceration causes pulmonary hematomas, traumatic pneumatoceles, and bronchopleural fistulae if they communicate with the pleural space.

- Pulmonary lacerations occur in both blunt and penetrating chest injuries and result from tearing and crushing of lung tissue from penetrating object (knife, bullet, rib), or shearing forces and tissue stresses that occur during chest compression.

- They can be deep within the lung or superficial and subpleural.

- Hemoptysis is very common.

- Radiographically, pulmonary lacerations are:
  - Usually round in shape, secondary to inherent lung elasticity, but can take days to form classic appearance; they become more evident on serial exams as surrounding pulmonary contusions clear
  - Usually 2 to 5 cm in diameter, though as large as 14 cm
  - Multiple or isolated; multiple usually secondary to compression injuries
  - +/– Air-containing, and, therefore, can have air/fluid levels
  - Usually present immediately after injury but often masked by pulmonary contusions, hemothorax, or pneumothorax

- Four types of lacerations are described on the basis of CT scan findings and mechanism of injury:
  - Compression rupture (most common)
  - Compression shear (often vertical and paravertebral)
  - Rib penetration (usually small)
  - Adhesion tears (rare)

- Pulmonary lacerations have little clinical significance other than as a marker of injury severity. However, detection of lacerations is important because they can become secondarily infected, and most importantly, can lead to prolonged chest tube drainage secondary to development of a bronchopleural fistula.

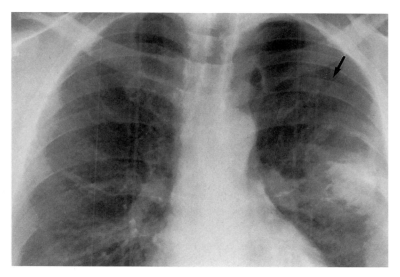

F I G U R E 2 3   AP chest radiograph from a 37-year-old-man involved in a motor-vehicle accident shows a large rounded opacity with an air/fluid level in the left mid-lung. Also note the left pneumothorax *(arrow)*, implying possible bronchopleural fistula. This is a pulmonary laceration probably related to sudden compression and direct lung rupture. Lacerations related to rib fractures are usually smaller.

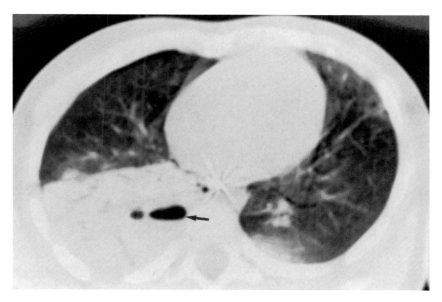

F I G U R E 2 4   CT scan from another patient involved in a motor-vehicle accident shows a Type II pulmonary laceration (compression-shear, paravertebral) in the right lung *(arrow),* with extensive surrounding lung contusion/atelectasis.

Suggested Reading

Wagner, R. B. et al. Classification of parenchymal injuries of the lung. *Radiology.* 1988;167: 77–82.

Pulmonary Laceration: Traumatic Pneumatocele (Stab Wound)

KEY FACTS

- The pulmonary laceration is present immediately after injury, but hemothorax or pneumothorax can obscure the underlying lung injury; the laceration becomes evident after satisfactory chest tube drainage.

- As in blunt trauma, pulmonary laceration due to a stab wound causes pulmonary hematomas, traumatic pneumatoceles, and bronchopleural fistulae.

- It can take days to for the classic appearance of a traumatic pneumatocele to appear. Look for a thin-walled, rounded lucency, usually 2 to 5 cm, depending upon the size of the knife.

- If blood fills the laceration instead of air, the laceration will be more mass-like (a hematoma).

- Simple pneumatoceles heal more quickly than hematomas.

- Stab wounds do not usually have associated pulmonary contusion, whereas a gunshot wound track is surrounded by a zone of contusion of variable size.

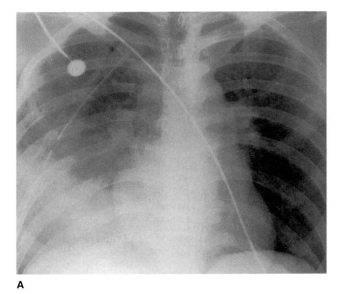

A

FIGURE 25   (A) An initial AP chest radiograph from a 20-year-old-man with a stab wound to the right chest wall shows a large right hemothorax. The underlying lung shows no apparent injury; the hemothorax obscures the pulmonary laceration.

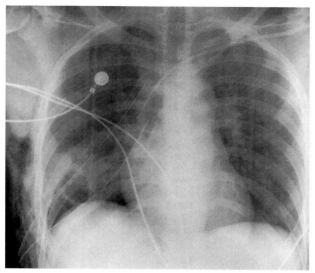

B

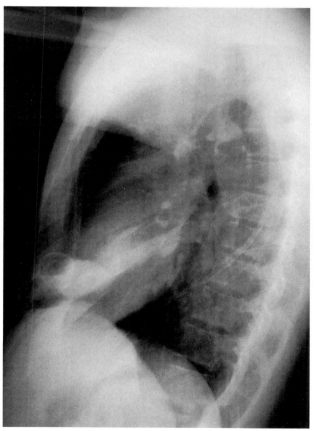

C

FIGURE 25   **(B), (C)** PA and lateral chest radiographs several days later show interval clearing of the hemothorax. Now evident is the elliptical shaped pulmonary laceration along the stabwound track. Note the air/fluid level on the lateral projection.

Suggested Reading

Groskin, S. *Radiological, Clinical and Biomechanical Aspects of Chest Trauma.* Berlin: Springer Verlag; 1991.

Pulmonary Laceration: Pulmonary Hematoma

KEY FACTS

- Pulmonary hematoma results from extensive hemorrhage into a pulmonary laceration. The clot undergoes typical organization and can have a fibrous wall, hence they become progressively opaque over time.

- Several weeks after an injury, a pulmonary hematoma can begin to appear as, and can be confused with, a solitary pulmonary nodule. However, they usually resolve spontaneously and are sometimes called vanishing lung tumors.

- Pulmonary hematomas can take weeks or months to heal, sometimes with substantial lung scarring.

- Occasionally, pulmonary hematomas form an air crescent sign and can be confused with a mycetoma.

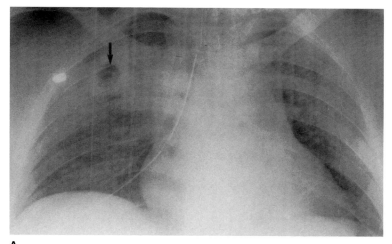

FIGURE 26 **(A)** AP chest radiograph from an 24-year-old-woman with a gunshot wound to the right chest shows a rounded lucency with surrounding opacity (zone of contusion) consistent with a pulmonary laceration in the right upper lobe *(arrow)*. **(B)** PA chest radiograph from the same patient, 6 weeks after initial injury, shows a spiculated mass at the site of the previous gunshot wound *(arrow)*. This represents a healing hematoma that can simulate a lung neoplasm.

Suggested Reading
Groskin, S. *Radiological, Clinical and Biomechanical Aspects of Chest Trauma*. Berlin: Springer Verlag; 1991.

Foreign Body Embolization and Retrieval

KEY FACTS

- The final location of an intravascular foreign body depends upon the type of object, size, material stiffness, site of entry, and position of the patient at the time of the accident. Blood flow patterns also play a key role. Most bullet emboli will follow the direction of flow, although 15% of venous bullet emboli cause embolization in a retrograde manner.

- An intravascular destination most often results from small-caliber, low-velocity bullets and shotgun pellets because they are less likely to penetrate both walls of a blood vessel. Peripheral venous foreign bodies (e.g., bullets, shotgun pellets, fragmented central lines), unless attached to the vein wall, embolize centrally.

- An intravascular bullet should be suspected when there is no exit wound and the missile is not identified within the expected path of the wound, or when serial radiographs demonstrate bullet migration. Arteriography and venography precisely localize the intravascular foreign body.

- Intravascular bullet emboli can produce infection, ischemia, or injury to organs or extremity distant from the site of injury. Bullet emboli to the heart are complicated by endocarditis, valvular dysfunction, and paradoxical emboli.

- Bullets within an artery are symptomatic in 80% of the cases, while bullets in the venous system are symptomatic in only one-third of patients. Arterial and venous bullet emboli not causing symptoms should be removed according to the risk of possible displacement and further embolization. Intraarterial bullet fragments that are likely to embolize to a critical location need to be removed as soon as possible. Bullet fragments (e.g., BB size) and catheter fragments (e.g., 1–2 cm) embolizing to the pulmonary vasculature may be left in place.

- Metallic foreign bodies that are smooth and intact, and catheter fragments, can be retrieved percutaneously by an interventional radiologist with the aid of snares, baskets, and grasping forceps. If unsuccessful, then surgical removal is often necessary. Jagged and deformed missiles require surgical removal.

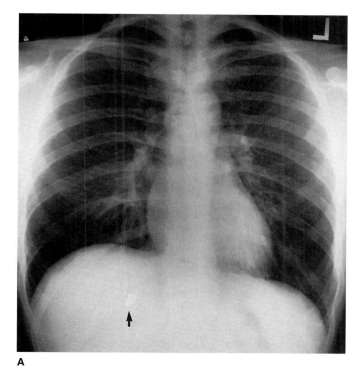

A

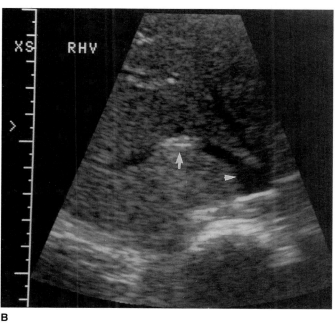

B

F I G U R E   2 7   9-year-old boy shot in the right anterior axillary line at sixth to seventh rib space with no exit wound. Admission chest radiograph (not shown) showed a bullet lying in the midline at the level of the T9 vertebral body. At laporatomy, there was a focal laceration of the anterior wall of the inferior vena cava. Post-operative chest radiograph **(A)** showed the bullet *(black arrow)* had migrated and was now located in right upper quadrant of abdomen. Ultrasonography **(B)** localized the bullet in the right hepatic vein *(white arrow)*, about 2 to 3 cm from the inferior vena cava *(white arrowhead).* Angiographic retrieval *(continued)*

Foreign Body Embolization and Retrieval
(Continued)

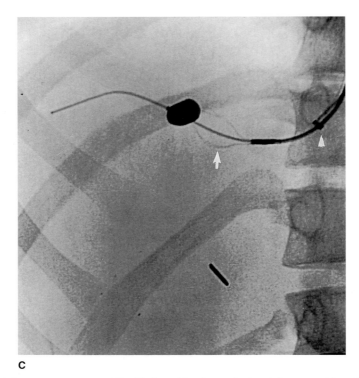

C

F I G U R E   2 7 (CONTINUED)   **(C)** of bullet with a Segura basket *(white arrow)* introduced via right internal jugular vein (white arrowhead is tip of vascular sheath).

Suggested Reading
Egglin TK, Dickey KW, Rosenblatt M, Pollak JS. Retrieval of intravascular foreign bodies: experience in 32 cases. *AJR.* 1995;164(5):1259–64.

Lung Injury: Blast Effect

KEY FACTS

- Blast effect itself can also cause injury to the lung, usually focal or diffuse pulmonary contusions that can be life-threatening. These types of pulmonary contusions are often more central in locations, unlike those associated with blunt chest wall injuries.

- Other injuries to the chest related to primary blast effect include pneumothorax and alveolar rupture with air embolism (leading to early death).

- Significant lung injury is proportional to the auditory injury and the blast force.

- In patients with flail chest (see Figure 3) and underlying pulmonary contusion, it is the contusion that is frequently the primary cause of hypoxia and morbidity.

- Lobar contusions after high velocity (assault/military weapons) gunshot wounds can lead to refractory hypoxemia. Contused lung loses autoregulation and literally shunts blood to itself, away from more normal lung (an intrapulmonary shunt). This type of severe lobar contusion can be treated with lobectomy.

- Shotgun pellets are considered low velocity projectiles, however, at close range there is a large blast effect and massive soft-tissue injury that can compromise the structural and mechanical integrity of the chest wall.

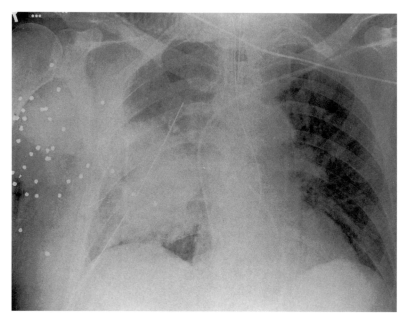

FIGURE 28   AP chest radiograph from a 69-year-old-man with a shotgun wound to the right chest wall. Note the extensive soft-tissue injury. Also, there is a large parenchymal opacity representing blast effect (pulmonary contusion).

Suggested Reading

Groskin, S. *Radiological, Clinical and Biomechanical Aspects of Chest Trauma*. Berlin: Springer Verlag; 1991.

Barotrauma

K E Y   F A C T S

- Barotrauma, or extra-alveolar, intra or extrathoracic air, has multiple etiologies:
  - Blunt or penetrating chest trauma with lung or GI tract injuries
  - Foreign body in upper or lower airways
  - Iatrogenic injuries to the airways or GI tract
  - Fractures of facial bones
  - Dental extractions and other oral surgical procedures
  - Infection by gas-producing organism
  - Air from outside body (penetrating trauma or surgery)
  - Mechanical ventilation
- Radiographically, disruption of the pulmonary parenchyma and airways can cause:
  - Pulmonary interstitial emphysema
  - Pneumothorax
  - Pneumomediastinum
  - Pneumatoceles
  - Pneumopericardium (rare)
- In severe cases of barotrauma, air can dissect from the mediastinum to the neck, face, chest, and abdominal wall, and retroperitoneum.

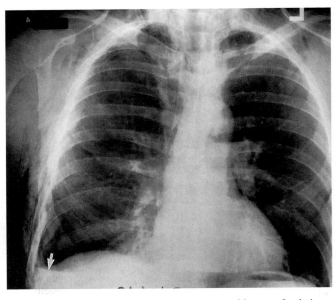

F I G U R E   2 9   Upright AP chest radiograph from a 43-year-old-man, after being assaulted, shows extensive subcutaneous emphysema, pneumomediastinum, and right hydropneumothorax *(arrow),* all resulting from rib fractures (not evident on this exam).

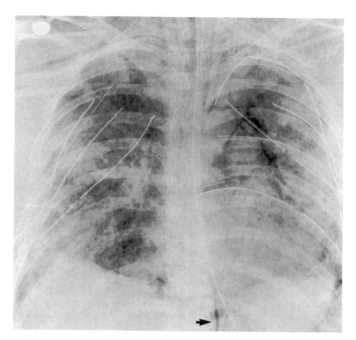

FIGURE 30 Supine AP chest radiograph from a 35-year-old-man involved in a high-speed boat accident shows diffuse parenchymal opacities consistent with adult respiratory distress syndrome. Positive pressure mechanical ventilation led to extensive barotrauma (extraalveolar air), including the "V-sign of Naclerio" *(arrow)*. This represents pneumomediastinum extending to the parietal pleura that covers the left hemidiaphragm.

Suggested Reading

Maunder RJ, Pierson DJ, Hudson LD. Subcutaneous and mediastinal emphysema: Pathophysiology, diagnosis, and management. *Arch Intern Med.* 1984;144:1447–1453.

Aspiration of Foreign Body

KEY FACTS

- Most common substances to be aspirated in trauma patients are food/vomitus, teeth, and road debris.
- In non-trauma patients, especially children, frequently aspirated foreign-bodies include coins, nuts, and small toys, most of which are radio-opaque.
- Distribution is as would be expected for any aspiration in the supine patient: dependent lung segments, namely the basal segmental bronchi of the lower lobes, superior segemental bronchi, and the apical-posterior segements of the upper lobes.
- Larger objects lodge in the central airways, while smaller objects can be seen at the periphery of the lung.
- Removal of intrabronchial teeth should be done expeditiously to avoid bronchial stenosis and obstructive pneumonitis.

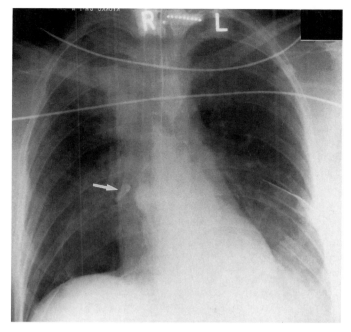

FIGURE 31 AP chest radiograph from a 20-year-old-man involved in a motor-vehicle accident shows a tooth in the right bronchus intermedius *(arrow)*. This must be retrieved, usually bronchoscopically, to avoid chronic obstruction and infection.

Suggested Reading
Limper AH, Prakash UB. Tracheobronchial foreign bodies in adults. *Ann Intern Med* 1990; 112:604–609.

Near-drowning

KEY FACTS

- Two prominent components of near-drowning are cerebral anoxia and pulmonary aspiration of water, the volume aspirated being more important than the nature of the fluid (fresh versus salt water).

- Radiographic assessment of near-drowning victims may vary greatly, ranging from a completely normal appearance to varying degrees of pulmonary edema.

- Important mechanisms of pulmonary edema appear to be loss of functional pulmonary surfactant, osmotically-driven influx of plasma after salt-water aspiration, and activation of inflammatory mediators with resultant diffuse alveolar damage and pulmonary capillary leakage.

- There may be a delay of 24 to 48 hours before pulmonary edema develops or the edema may be present initially and resolve very rapidly, even within hours.

- In most instances there is marked clearing of the lungs within 3 to 5 days, with complete resolution of pulmonary edema within 7 to 10 days.

- In a near-drowning patient, scuba diving further increases the risks of developing lung barotrauma and decompression sickness.

- Mild decompression sickness (Type I): symptoms relate to the formation of periarticular soft-tissue gas bubbles (the "bends").

- Severe decompression sickness (Type II): direct transit of inert molecular gas into the pulmonary or systemic arterial circulations ("gas embolism") may result in pulmonary insufficiency (the "chokes") or central nervous signs and symptoms. Severe decompression sickness, especially with cerebral gas embolism, always requires urgent hyperbaric therapy.

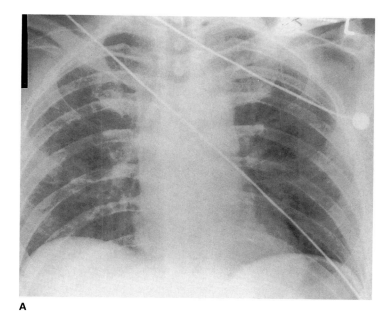

A

B

F I G U R E   3 2   **(A)** 40-year-old-man suffered near-drowning while scuba diving at a depth of 40 feet. Initial chest radiograph shows diffuse parenchymal opacities consistent with pulmonary edema. **(B)** Chest radiograph obtained 9 hours after **(A),** and after hyperbaric oxygen therapy, shows complete resolution of pulmonary edema.

Suggested Reading

Hunter TB, Whitehouse WM. Fresh-water near-drowning: Radiological aspects. *Radiology.* 1974;112:51–56.

Intraperitoneal Fluid in Trauma

K E Y   F A C T S

- Intraperitoneal fluid in an acutely traumatized patient represents one or more of the following:
  - Blood (rarely with intravascular contrast)
  - Intestinal fluid (+/− oral contrast)
  - Urine
  - Bile
  - Lymphatic fluid
  - Diagnostic lavage fluid
  - Preexisting ascites
- The attenuation of fluid, as measured on CT scan in Hounsfield units (HU), can indicate its origin. Bowel contents (without oral contrast), urine, bile, lavage fluid, and preexisting ascites measure near water density (<20 HU).
- Clotted blood generally measures 45 to 75 HU; but prior to clot formation, following clot lysis, and in the anemic or aggressively hydrated patient, the attenuation of hemoperitoneum will be lower, 25 to 50 HU or less.
- High attenuation peritoneal fluid (>100 HU) indicates extraluminal oral contrast due to bowel perforation, or, rarely, active extravasation of contrast-laden blood from a vascular injury.
- Blood remains higher in attenuation near its site of origin. A higher attenuation (45 to 75 HU) localized hematoma *(sentinel clot)* can help localize the source of hemoperitoneum.
- Separation of the high attenuation clot from low attenuation serum *(hematocrit effect)* can occur within hours; this finding confirms hemoperitoneum.
- Fluid between loops of bowel *(interloop fluid)* suggests bowel or mesenteric injury, even following diagnostic peritoneal lavage (DPL). Perforation is suggested by water attenuation fluid or oral contrast. Intermediate attenuation interloop fluid (25–50 HU) is usually a mesenteric hematoma.
- Patients with small quantities of intraperitoneal fluid or a small mesenteric hematoma as the sole abnormality on CT scan, if otherwise clinically stable, may be able to be managed conservatively.

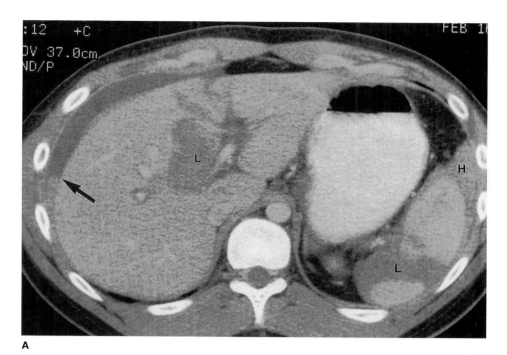

A

F I G U R E 3 3   CT scan of hemoperitoneum. **(A)** Contrast-enhanced CT scan in a young adult male who sustained blunt abdominal trauma. There are lacerations of liver and spleen (L) with adjacent hemoperitoneum. The blood adjacent to the liver shows a hematocrit effect *(arrow)*. The dense hematoma (H) adjacent to the spleen indicates the spleen is one of the sources of hemoperitoneum. *(continued)*

Intraperitoneal Fluid in Trauma (Continued)

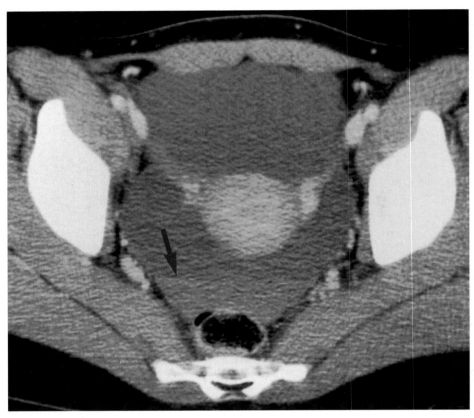

B

FIGURE 33 (CONTINUED)   **(B)** Young adult woman with hemoperitoneum in pelvis showing
hematocrit effect *(arrow).*

Suggested Reading

Levine CD, Patel UJ, Wachsberg RH, Simmons MZ, Baker SR, Cho KC. CT in patients with
   blunt abdominal trauma: Clinical significance of intraperitoneal fluid detected on a scan
   with otherwise normal findings. *AJR.* 1995;164:1381–1385.

Levine CD, Patel UJ, Silverman PM, Wachsberg RH. Low attenuation of acute traumatic
   hemoperitoneum on CT scans. *AJR.* 1996;166:1089–1093.

Extraperitoneal Fluid in Trauma

KEY FACTS

- CT scanning is the primary modality for evaluating retroperitoneal trauma.

- The anterior pararenal space contains the pancreas and the retroperitoneal parts of the duodenum, ascending colon, and descending colon. It is a common location for fluid to accumulate following abdominal trauma.

- Fasciae are often disrupted by trauma, therefore, retroperitoneal fluid collections may not be rigidly limited by well-known fascial planes.

- Focal fluid collections adjacent to a retroperitoneal segment of bowel may indicate focal bowel injury, including perforation.

- Large quantities of retroperitoneal fluid, without solid organ injury, may be due to a major vascular injury in retroperitoneum or mesenteric root.

- Blood can dissect upward into the abdominal retroperitoneum from pelvic fractures and associated vascular injuries.

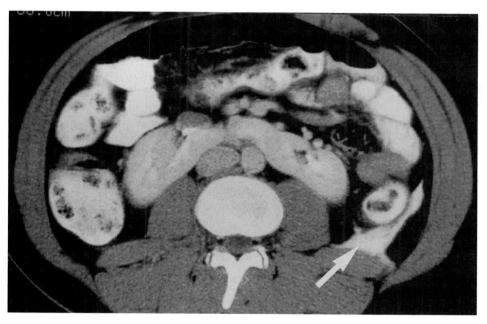

FIGURE 34   CT scan of retroperitoneal fluid. Young adult male who sustained a knife wound to left flank. Oral, rectal, and intravenous contrast have been administered. There is extraluminal contrast in the left anterior pararenal space indicating an extraperitoneal colon laceration *(arrow)*. Note the horseshoe kidney.

Suggested Reading

Korobkin et al. CT of the extraperitoneal space: Normal anatomy and fluid collections. *AJR.* 1992;159:933–941.

Intraperitoneal and Retroperitoneal Gas

KEY FACTS

- In trauma, pneumoperitoneum and retroperitoneal gas can originate from a perforated viscus, a penetrating wound, or peritoneal lavage. Retroperitoneal gas can also originate from intrathoracic injuries resulting in pneumothorax or pneumomediastinum with air dissecting through fascial planes into the abdomen.

- Computed tomography is the most sensitive modality for detecting small quantities of free intraperitoneal gas, particularly in the acutely traumatized patient who must remain supine. Look for it in the most non-dependent portion of the peritoneal cavity using wide (lung) windows.

- The presence of non-dependent intraperitoneal gas is nonspecific if the patient has had a peritoneal lavage or recent abdominal surgery. Gas trapped within dependent areas of the peritoneum, particularly between leaves of mesenteries, suggests bowel perforation in the acute setting and abscess formation later.

- The presence of a focal retroperitoneal gas collection near a retroperitoneal segment of a hollow viscus (duodenum, ascending colon, descending colon, rectum) at CT scanning suggests a retroperitoneal hollow viscus injury. Note however, a gas-containing diverticulum, a relatively common finding of the retroperitoneal duodenum, can simulate a solitary retroperitoneal gas bubble.

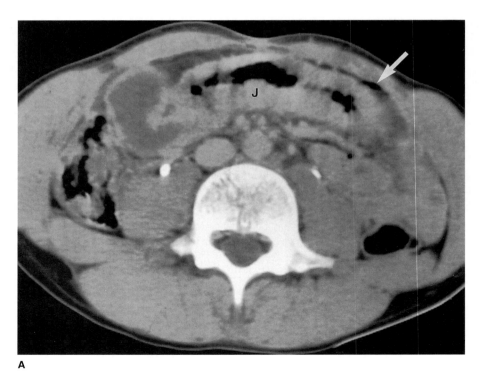

A

F I G U R E   3 5   Intra and extraperitoneal gas on CT scan. **(A)** Young male following a motor-vehicle accident. The thick-walled jejunum (J) and bubble of intraperitoneal gas *(arrow)* indicate jejunal perforation.

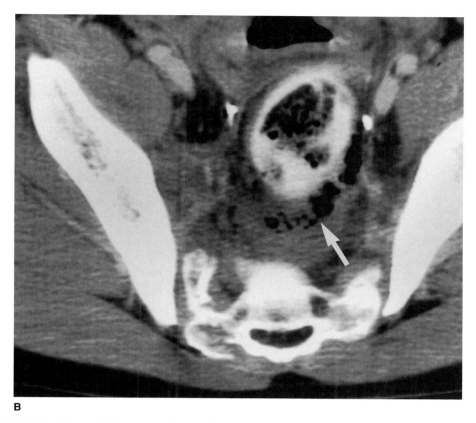

B

FIGURE 35   **(B)** Young male involved in a motorcycle collision. Perirectal air and fluid *(arrow)* are due to a rectal perforation.

Suggested Reading

Hamilton P, Rizoli S, McLellan B, Murphy J. Significance of intra-abdominal extraluminal air detected by CT scan in blunt abdominal trauma. *J Trauma.* 1995;39:331–333.

Active Bleeding: Findings on CT Scan

KEY FACTS

- Contrast-enhanced CT scan can detect active bleeding. Dynamic incremental, or spiral CT scanning with intravascular contrast enhancement is essential to depict active extravasation.

- In children, active bleeding is most often seen associated with solid organ injury, particularly the spleen and liver. In adults, the iliac vessels (associated with pelvic fractures) are the most frequent sites of active bleeding, however, the spleen, liver, and kidney are also common sites.

- The primary finding on CT scan is a focal dense collection of contrast-enhanced blood, always associated with a surrounding hematoma. CT scan attenuation of actively extravasating contrast-enhanced blood usually ranges from 85 to 370 (mean 132) HU.

- Bleeding into the peritoneal cavity results in layering or incomplete mixing of contrast-enhanced blood and nonenhanced intraperitoneal fluid.

- The site of extravasation identified on CT scan corresponds closely with the actual bleeding vessel. This information facilitates the initial approach in selective angiographic embolization.

- Indicators of shock and hypovolemia include:
  - Flattened IVC
  - Small aorta and mesenteric vessels
  - Persistent nephrogram without excretion
  - Thickened small bowel folds
  - Small, hypoattenuating spleen

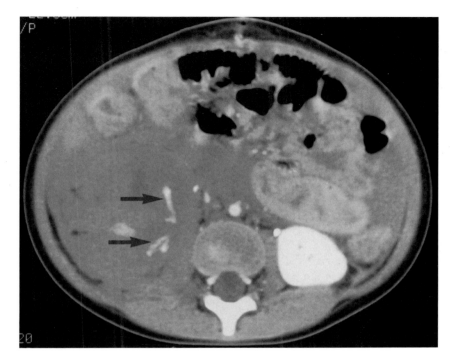

FIGURE 36   Two high-attenuation contrast collections *(arrows)* due to active arterial bleeding into a large perinephric hematoma from a renal vascular pedicle injury.

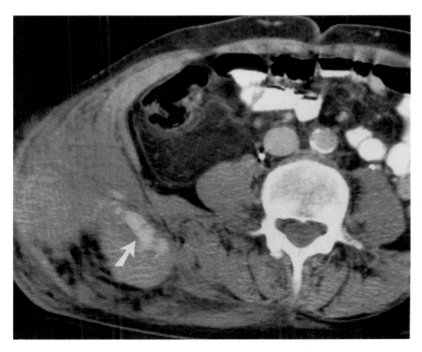

FIGURE 37   High attenuation contrast-laden blood *(arrow)* in a flank hematoma secondary to injury of a lumbar artery.

Suggested Reading

Shanmuganathan K, Mirvis SE, Sover ER. Value of contrast-enhanced CT in detecting active hemorrhage in patients with blunt abdominal or pelvic trauma. *AJR.* 1993;161:65–69.

Liver Injury: Overview

KEY FACTS

- In patients with blunt abdominal trauma, the liver is a frequently injured organ within the abdomen, second only to the spleen. The right lobe is more commonly injured than the left lobe. Isolated injuries carry a low mortality, but this increases significantly when the liver injury is associated with multiple other injuries.

- Right hepatic lobe injuries are associated with rib fractures, adrenal hematomas, and lung and renal contusions, while left hepatic lobe injuries are associated with pancreatic, duodenal, and colonic injuries.

- Contrast-enhanced CT scan is the modality of choice for the evaluation of liver injuries in the hemodynamically stable patient.

- Hepatic injuries can be categorized based on their CT scan appearance;
  - Lacerations—either simple (linear) or complex (stellate)
  - Fractures—through-and-through parenchymal lacerations that may result in avulsion of a portion of the liver
  - Contusions—areas of low-attenuation parenchymal hemotoma
  - Hematomas—either subcapsular peripheral lentiform collections, or irregular high-attenuation intraparenchymal collections of blood

- CT scan grading of liver injuries (from Ralls, Recommended Reading, below):

    I. Capsular tears and lacerations < 1 cm

    II. Lacerations 1 to 3 cm

    III. Subcapsular hematomas < 10 cm, deep or stellate fractures

    IV. Large subcapsular hematomas, extensive parenchymal damage

    V. Crush injuries with bilobar damage, avulsion hepatic vein injuries

- There is a growing tendency to operate based on a patient's clinical status rather than CT scan findings. High grade injuries can be managed non-surgically if the patient remains clinically and hemodynamically stable.

- Artifacts on CT scans that can simulate a liver laceration:
    - Streak artifact off of air-fluid level or nasogastric tube in stomach
    - Beam hardening from ribs or patient's arms
    - Focal fatty infiltration

- Hints on CT scanning technique in abdominal trauma:
    - Pull the nasogastric tube back into esophagus before scanning
    - Remove metallic leads (e.g., ECG leads) from scanning field
    - Put the patient's arms overhead
    - If patient is mechanically ventilated, suspend ventilation during scanning

Liver Injury: Overview *(Continued)*

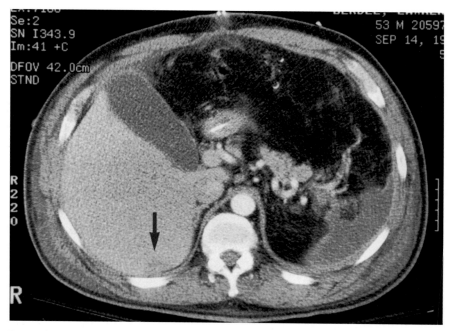

FIGURE 38   Subtle Grade I liver laceration *(arrow)* in the posterior right lobe.

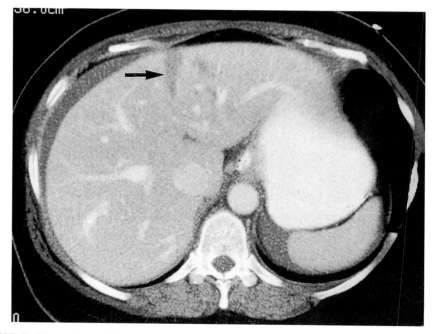

FIGURE 39   Grade II liver laceration *(arrow)* extends approximately 3 cm deep to the capsule.

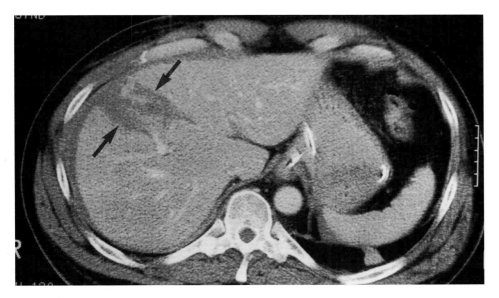

F I G U R E   4 0   Deep Grade III liver laceration extending toward hilum *(arrows)*.

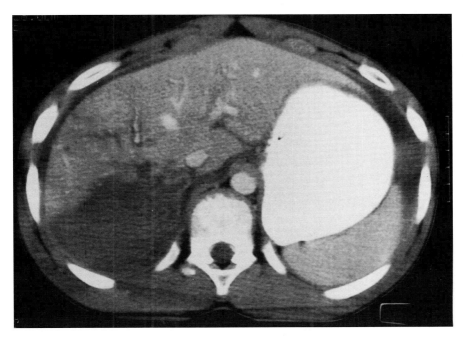

F I G U R E   4 1   Grade IV liver laceration with devascularization of posterior right hepatic lobe.

Suggested Reading

Ralls PW. The liver. In: Jeffrey RB, Ralls PW. eds. *CT and Sonography of the Acute Abdomen.* 2nd ed. Philadelphia: Lippincott-Raven; 1996.

Liver Injury: Natural History

KEY FACTS

- Non-surgical management of liver injuries in hemodynamically stable patients is now widely accepted. This has lead to an understanding of the natural healing process following traumatic liver injury.

- Follow-up CT scan frequently demonstrates marked decrease in the size of parenchymal hematomas and lacerations within the first week following injury.

- Most intraperitoneal fluid resorbs within 3 to 7 days. If the volume of fluid is unchanged or has increased on a follow-up examination, continued bleeding or bile leakage should be considered. Demonstration of expanding hematoma or active hemorrhage warrants angiographic or surgical evaluation.

- Discrete fluid collections such as bilomas and liquified hematomas can be followed with ultrasound.

- Delayed complications occur in up to 10% to 20% of patients with traumatic liver injury treated non-operatively. These complications are frequently detected on follow-up CT scan examinations and include:

  - Recurrent hemorrhage; usually noted in first several days

  - Biloma and other biliary injuries (see following section)

  - Infection of an intrahepatic hematoma or biloma, especially following penetrating injury

  - Pseudoaneurysm formation

  - Arteriovenous fistula

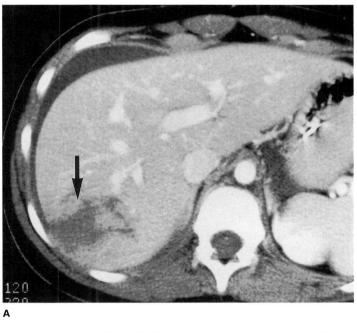

A

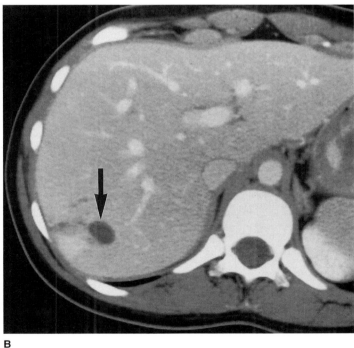

B

F I G U R E   4 2   **(A)** Grade III right hepatic hematoma *(arrow)* managed conservatively in a hemodynamically stable patient. **(B)** Follow-up CT scan demonstrates substantial decrease in size of the hematoma and laceration *(arrow)* as well as resolution of hemoperitoneum.

Suggested Reading

Harris LM, Booth FV, Hassett JM Jr. Liver lacerations—A marker of severe but sometimes subtle intra-abdominal injuries in adults. *J Trauma*. 1991;31:894–899.

Biliary Injury

KEY FACTS

- Both the intra- and extrahepatic biliary system may be injured in patients with blunt or penetrating abdominal trauma.

- Intrahepatic biliary injury is usually caused by a liver laceration that disrupts the biliary tree. Biliary injuries are often found incidentally on follow-up examination.

- A biloma is a collection of bile outside the biliary system. The bile may be contained as an intrahepatic cyst, or may form a collection within the peritoneum.

- Most post-traumatic bilomas resolve spontaneously without intervention or surgery. Bilomas causing pain or obstruction or those that become infected are treated by guided aspiration or by catheter drainage.

- Injury to the liver and biliary system may also lead to:
    - Hemobilia—due to communication between a vascular structure (usually hepatic arterial branch) and the biliary tree
    - Jaundice—an enlarging subcapsular hematoma can exert a compressive effect on central biliary ducts adequate to cause obstructive jaundice
    - Bilehemia—leakage of bile into the systemic venous system

- Trauma to the gallbladder is rare. CT scan findings with traumatic gallbladder rupture include a contracted or nonvisualized gallbladder and intraperitoneal low attenuation bile. Patients can be surprisingly asymptomatic. With avulsion of the gallbladder pedicle, patients will typically have a large hematoma in the gallbladder bed with hemoperitoneum and bile ascites.

- Radionuclide biliary (HIDA) scan and percutaneous transhepatic cholangiography (PTC) can be useful to show persistent intraperitoneal bile leaks.

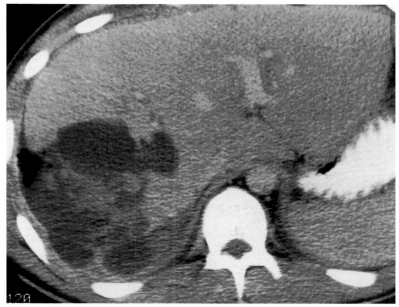

A

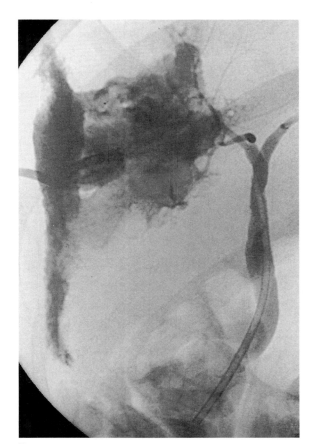

FIGURE 43

Complicated post-traumatic biloma. **(A)** CT scan demonstrates low attenuation fluid in the posterior right hepatic lobe. **(B)** Cholangiogram performed via a drainage catheter demonstrates communication with the central biliary tree as well as free intaperitoneal leakage. The patient was successfully managed with percutaneous catheter drainage and internal stenting.

B

Suggested Reading

Ralls PW. The gallbladder and bile ducts. In: Jeffrey RB, Ralls, PW, eds. *CT and Sonography of the Acute Abdomen*. 2nd ed. Philadelphia: Lippincott-Raven; 1996.

Splenic Trauma

KEY FACTS

- The spleen is the most frequently injured abdominal organ in blunt abdominal trauma. Left lower rib fractures, left upper quadrant pain, and hemodynamic instability can be seen with splenic injury. Contrast-enhanced CT scan is approximately 95% sensitive and specific for detection of splenic injury.

- Splenic injuries include subcapsular and intraparenchymal hematomas, lacerations, fractures, and vascular pedicle injuries.

- Perisplenic fluid collections are the only sign of splenic injury in 15% to 20% of cases. The sentinel clot sign, in which the attenuation of hemoperitoneum is highest adjacent to the injured organ, is a reliable predictor of splenic trauma.

- CT scan grading of splenic injuries:

    I. Localized capsular disruption; small subcapsular hematoma

    II. Small parenchymal laceration; parenchymal hematoma <3 cm

    III. Fractures extending to hilum; parenchymal hematomas >3 cm

    IV. Shattered spleen; vascular disruption

- CT scan accurately grades splenic injuries, but does not allow accurate prediction of which patients may be successfully managed nonoperatively. Some patients with high grade injuries can be successfully managed nonsurgically, while other patients with low grade injuries will fail conservative management.

- In children, nonoperative treatment is well established. In adults, the therapeutic approach seems to be evolving toward splenic salvage whenever possible, rather than splenectomy. Splenic preservation prevents postsplenectomy sepsis.

- Congenital clefts are usually seen on the medial aspect of the spleen, these may be confused with small lacerations which are usually seen on the lateral aspect.

- Delayed rupture is defined as active splenic hemorrhage that occurs 48 hours or more following injury. The incidence of delayed rupture has decreased dramatically in recent years with improvements in imaging and clinical monitoring techniques.

- Other potential pitfalls in splenic injury evaluation:
    - Streak artifact from adjacent ribs
    - Heterogeneous enhancement on spiral CT scan images obtained prior to the portal-venous phase
    - Diffusely hypodense spleen associated with hypovolemic shock

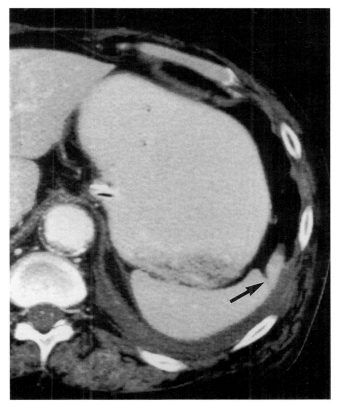

F I G U R E 4 4   Normal splenic cleft *(arrow)* should not be mistaken for a laceration.

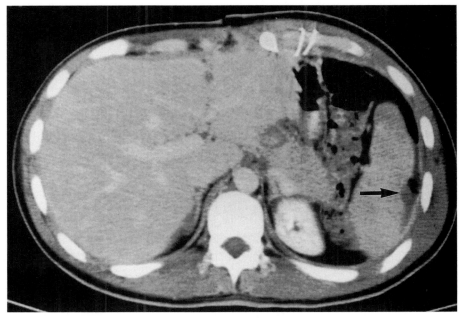

F I G U R E 4 5   Localized capsular disruption (Grade I) with small subcapsular hematoma *(arrow)*.

Splenic Trauma *(Continued)*

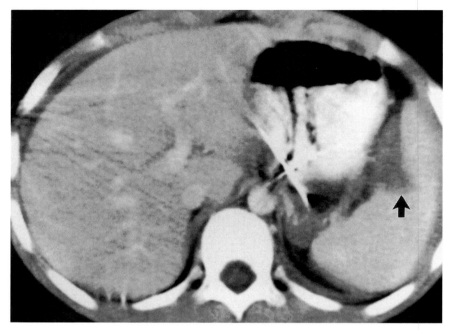

F I G U R E   4 6   Parenchymal laceration and 3 cm hematoma seen along medial aspect of spleen *(arrow).*

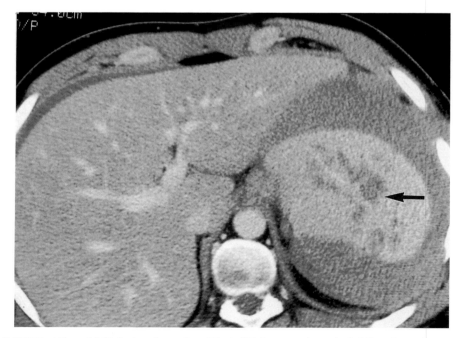

F I G U R E   4 7   Multiple deep lacerations (Grade III) that extend to splenic hilum *(arrow).*

Section 2: Imaging Fundamentals

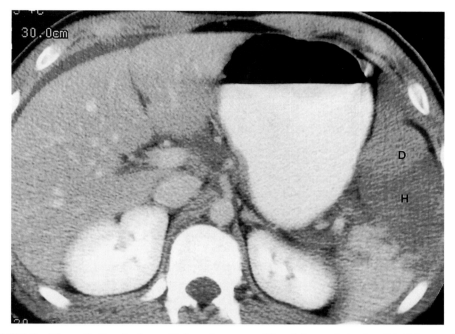

F I G U R E   4 8   Shattered spleen with large hematoma (H) and devascularization (D) of the anterior segment.

Suggested Reading

Raptopoulos V. Abdominal trauma. Emphasis on computed tomography. *Radiol Clin North Am.* 1994;32:969–987.

Kluger Y, Paul DB, Raves JJ, et al. Delayed rupture of the spleen—myths, facts, and their importance: Case reports and literature review. *J Trauma.* 1994;36:568–571.

Pancreatic Injury

KEY FACTS

- The deep retroperitoneal location of the pancreas provides relative protection from injury. Therefore, pancreatic injuries are much less common than liver or spleen injuries.

- Penetrating injury is 3 to 4 times more common than blunt injury. A blow to the epigastrium is the usual etiology: steering wheels in adults, handlebars in children, and child abuse in infants.

- There are associated visceral (most often liver or spleen) injuries in up to 90%.

- The most common site of pancreatic laceration is the pancreatic neck.

- Injury to the pancreatic duct and delay in diagnosis result in increased morbidity and mortality.

- Most pancreatic injuries are discovered during emergent laparotomy for intraperitoneal visceral or vascular injuries.

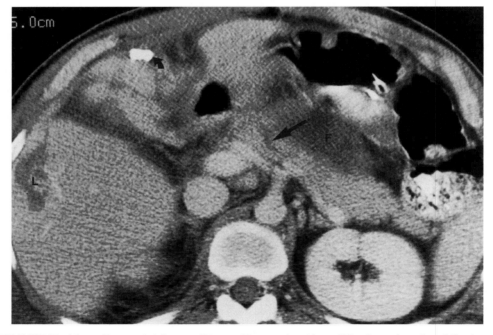

FIGURE 49   Pancreatic injury on CT scan. Young male with a mildly elevated amylase following exploratory laparotomy for injuries sustained in a motor-vehicle accident. There is a linear area of decreased attenuation at the pancreatic neck *(straight arrow)* and a lesser sac fluid collection (F); these indicate a pancreatic laceration. Note that there is also a liver laceration (L) and a surgical drain has been placed *(curved arrow).*

- CT scan may have sensitivities and specificities as high as 80% for pancreatic injury, but sensitivity may be as low as 60% in the first 12 hours following injury. If the clinical suspicion for pancreatic injury remains high, a repeat scan may be warranted.

- CT scan findings include:

  - Linear low attenuation area (laceration or transection)

  - Pancreatic enlargement or inhomogeneity

  - Peripancreatic fat stranding or fluid

  - Lesser sac fluid

  - Fluid between pancreas and splenic vein

- Endoscopic retrograde (ERCP) or intraoperative pancreatography may be used to establish pancreatic duct integrity.

- Complications of pancreatic trauma include pancreatitis, pseudocysts, and fistulae.

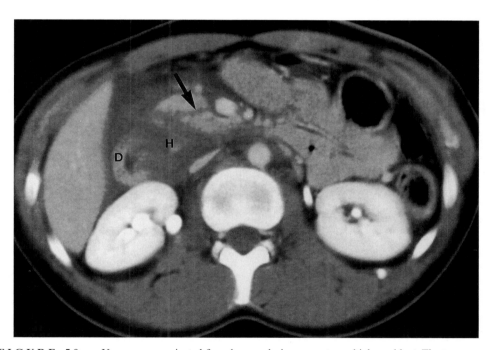

F I G U R E 5 0   Young woman ejected from her car during an motor-vehicle accident. The transverse lucency through the pancreatic uncinate *(arrow)* indicates a laceration. The pancreatic head has been avulsed from the duodenum (D) and a hematoma (H) separates the two structures. (Reproduced with permission from *AJR*. 1996;167:1152.) (From Fischer JH, et al. CT diagnosis of an isolated blunt pancreatic injury. *AJR* 1996;167:1152, with permission.)

Suggested Reading

Jurkovich GJ. Injuries to the duodenum and pancreas. In: Feliciano DV, Moore EE, Mattox KL, eds. *Trauma*. 3rd ed. Stamford: Appleton & Lange; 1996:573–594.

Gastrointestinal and Mesenteric Injury

KEY FACTS

- Gastrointestinal perforation is a surgical emergency. Bowel wall contusions can cause paralytic ileus while hematomas can cause obstruction.

- Mesenteric vascular injuries can cause segmental bowel ischemia or infarction. Large mesenteric tears can result in internal hernias.

- Patterns of bowel injury include:
  - Intraperitoneal hollow viscus injuries are more frequent than extraperitoneal bowel injuries
  - Injuries to the small bowel, colon, and stomach are relatively common in penetrating trauma
  - Hollow viscus injuries are less common in blunt trauma and usually involve the small bowel
  - Colon and gastric injuries are rare in blunt trauma
  - In blunt trauma small bowel injuries tend to occur near points of attachment: the ligament of Treitz and the ileocecal valve

- CT scan signs of intestinal or mesenteric injury:
  - Extralumenal oral contrast
  - Intraperitoneal air
  - Focal bowel wall thickening
  - Focal fluid collection (interloop fluid)
  - Focal dense hematoma (sentinel clot)
  - Substantial free intraperitoneal fluid without obvious solid organ injury

- Interloop fluid suggests bowel or mesenteric injury. Perforation results in extralumimal water-attenuation fluid or oral contrast. Intermediate attenuation interloop fluid (25–50 HU) is usually a mesenteric hematoma.

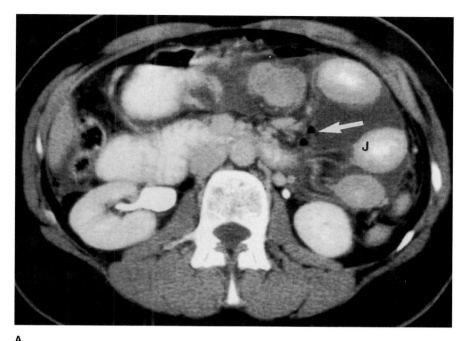

A

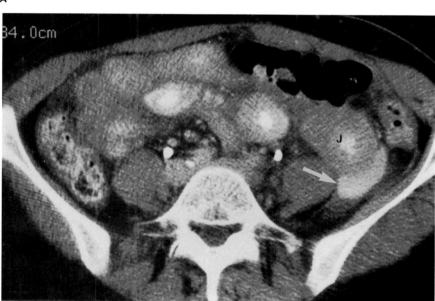

B

FIGURE 51   Jejunal perforation on CT scan. **(A)** Young woman with increasing abdominal pain 24 hours after a motor-vehicle accident (MVA). Thickened loops of jejunum (J) and interloop fluid and gas *(arrow)* indicate a jejunal perforation. **(B)** Middle-aged man involved in a head-on MVA. Jejunal wall thickening (J) and localized extraluminal oral contrast *(arrow)* indicate a jejunal perforation.

Suggested Reading
Orwig D, Federle MP. Localized clotted blood as evidence of visceral trauma on CT: The sentinel clot sign. *AJR*. 1989;153:747–749.

Duodenal Injury

KEY FACTS

- Duodenal perforation is a surgical emergency. Diagnostic delay results in increased morbidity and mortality. Duodenal hematoma, without perforation, can be treated conservatively.

- Penetrating injury is 3 to 4 times more common than blunt injury. A blow to the epigastrium is the usual etiology: steering wheels in adults, handlebars in children, and child abuse in infants.

- Associated pancreatic injuries are common.

- CT scan is the imaging modality of choice in blunt duodenal injury; CT can usually distinguish duodenal perforation from an isolated duodenal hematoma.

- CT scan findings of retroperitoneal duodenal injury:
  - Retroperitoneal gas near the duodenum
  - Focal paraduodenal fluid in the absence of diffuse retroperitoneal fluid
  - Focal duodenal wall thickening suggesting intramural hematoma

- Causes for a false-positive CT scan include:
  - Unopacified bowel loops adjacent to duodenum
  - Retroperitoneal hematoma from non-duodenal source
  - Duodenal diverticulum simulating retroperitoneal air

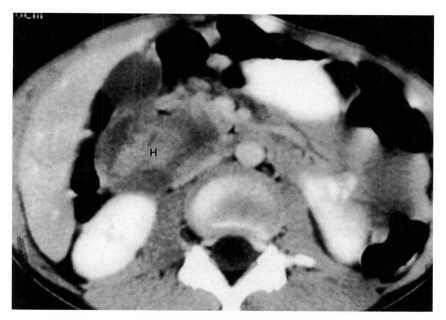

F I G U R E   5 2   Duodenal hematoma on CT scan. 7-year-old girl with a handle bar injury. Duodenal wall thickening with central high attenuation (H) indicates a duodenal hematoma.

Suggested Reading

Kunin JR, Korobkin M, Ellis JH, Francis IR, Kane NM, Siegel SE. Duodenal injuries caused by blunt abdominal trauma: Value of CT in differentiating perforation from hematoma. *AJR* 1993;160:1221–1223.

Extraperitoneal Colonic Injury

KEY FACTS

- The ascending and descending colon and rectum are covered by peritoneum only along their anterior surfaces therefore perforations in these areas are usually extraperitoneal.

- Rectal injuries occur in penetrating trauma and with blunt pelvic trauma associated with fractures.

- The ascending and descending colon are particularly at risk from stab and gunshot wounds to the flank.

- Diagnostic peritoneal lavage will be negative if injuries are isolated to the retroperitoneal portions of the colon. Therefore, CT scan with rectal contrast ("triple contrast") can be an important adjunct to DPL in patients with flank stab wounds and a negative DPL.

- CT scan signs of extraperitoneal colonic injury include anterior pararenal space gas or fluid and juxtacolonic fatty stranding. Any one of these findings warrants exploratory laparotomy in the setting of a penetrating flank injury.

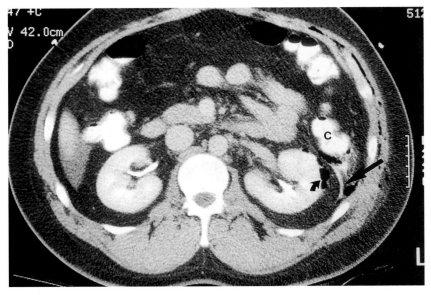

FIGURE 53   Descending colon laceration on "triple contrast" CT scan. Young man with a left flank stab wound and negative DPL. Gas and contrast have collected along the anterior renal fascia *(straight arrow)*, within the anterior pararenal space, indicating perforation of the descending colon (C). Note there is also gas beneath the left renal capsule *(curved arrow)*.

Suggested Reading

Hauser CJ, Huprich JE, Bosco P, Gibbons L, Mansour AY, Weiss AR. Triple-contrast computed tomography in the evaluation of penetrating posterior abdominal injuries. *Arch Surg* 1987;122:1112–1115.

Adrenal Hemorrhage

KEY FACTS

- Adrenal hemorrhage from blunt trauma is usually unilateral occurring on the right side twice as often as the left. Right-sided hemorrhage may be more common because of elevated venous pressures propagated from the adjacent IVC or because of compression by the liver.

- Adrenal hemorrhage is associated with ipsilateral abdominal or thoracic injuries in up to 95% of patients.

- Adrenal hemorrhage is usually of little clinical significance when unilateral. Large right sided hematomas can compress the IVC resulting in IVC thrombosis. Bilateral adrenal hemorrhages are uncommon, but can rarely result in adrenal insufficiency.

- On CT scan, adrenal hemorrhage usually appears as a discreet mass in the expected location of the adrenal gland. Less common patterns include diffuse enlargement of the adrenal without loss of the gland's normal shape and a cental mass displacing the adrenal limbs. The attenuation and heterogeneity of the hematoma will vary depending on its age. There is usually associated stranding of the adjacent fat.

- An isolated adrenal mass, without associated adjacent fatty stranding, requires follow up CT scan to exclude a neoplasm.

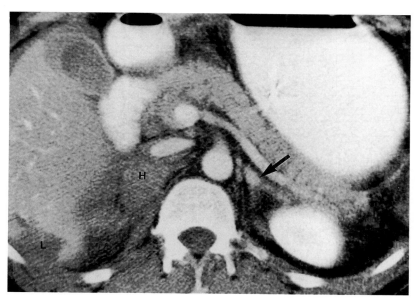

FIGURE 54   CT scan from a 32-year-old male involved in a motor-vehicle accident. There is an intermediate attenuation mass replacing the right adrenal gland indicating an adrenal hematoma (H). The left adrenal is normal *(arrow)*. There is an associated liver laceration (L).

Suggested Reading

Burks DW, Mirvis SE, Shanmuganathan K. Acute adrenal injury after blunt abdominal trauma: CT findings. *AJR.* 1992;158:503–507.

Renal Injuries

KEY FACTS

- The types of renal injuries from blunt trauma are:
  - Contusion
  - Laceration, with or without collecting system tear
  - Vascular pedicle laceration, occlusion or avulsion
  - Uretero-pelvic junction laceration or avulsion
- Grading system for renal injuries based on the Organ Injury Scaling (OIS) Committee of the American Association for the Surgery of Trauma (Note: all grading systems are generalizations; individual cases are sometimes difficult to fit exactly into a particular grade).
  - Grade 1: subcapsular, nonexpanding hematoma without laceration; contusion usually present
  - Grade 2: superficial laceration < 1.0 cm deep
  - Grade 3: laceration > 1.0 cm deep without collecting system rupture or urinary extravasation
  - Grade 4: laceration extending through renal cortex, medulla, and collecting system; or, main renal artery/vein injury with contained hemorrhage
  - Grade 5: shattered kidney; or, avulsion of renal hilum with totally infarcted kidney
  - 85% of renal injuries are Grade 1 or 2. Major renal injuries are Grades 3 to 5.

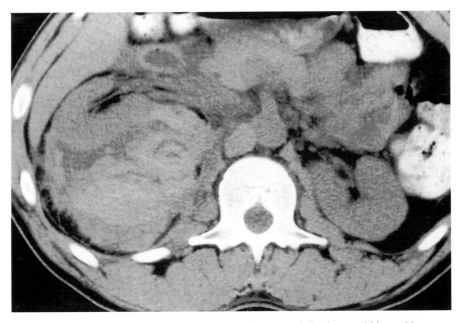

FIGURE 55   Large subcapsular and perinephric hematoma following renal biopsy. Noncontrast CT shows heterogeneous, high attenuation hematoma with "jelly roll" pattern. Hematoma displaces right kidney anteriorly and flattens posterior surface of parenchyma.

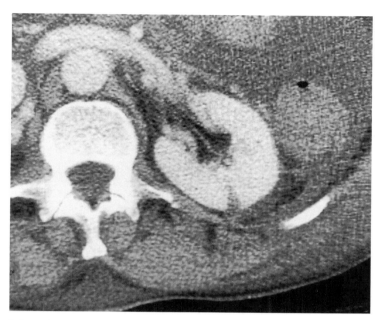

F I G U R E 5 6   Superficial renal laceration (Grade 2 injury). CT shows posterior, wedge-shaped nephrographic defect associated with small, localized perinephric hematoma.

Suggested Reading

Federle, MP. Evaluation of renal trauma. Chapter 51. In: Pollack HM, ed. *Clinical Urography: An Atlas and Textbook of Urological Imaging.* Philadelphia: WB Saunders; 1990:1472–1494.

Renal Injuries: Imaging

KEY FACTS

- The "one-shot" IVU is reserved for hemodynamically unstable patients who are being whisked to surgery. Most will have penetrating injuries.

- CT is the most accurate way to grade renal injuries; indicated in patients with blunt trauma who have gross hematuria, or microhematuria, plus hypotension. Twenty-five percent of such patients have a major (Grade 3 to 5) renal injury.

- CT scan findings:

  - Contusion (Grade 1): focal region(s) of diminished nephrogram; linear or patchy contrast "staining" of parenchyma on delayed images

  - Infarct: focal, geographic, sharply marginated nephrographic defect; cortical rim sign may be present, especially after several days

  - Acute subcapsular hematoma: crescentic, high attenuation blood collection over the renal surface; often flattens adjacent parenchyma; large perinephric hematoma often has a subcapsular component and may flatten and displace the kidney (Figure 55)

  - Superficial laceration (Grade 2): small linear or wedge shaped cortical nephrographic defect, often with focal perinephric or subcapsular hematoma (Figure 56)

  - Deep laceration (Grade 3): usually associated with moderate or large perinephric hematoma; collecting system intact

  - Deep laceration with tear of collecting system (Grade 4): extravasation of contrast-enhanced urine is pathognomonic; vascular phase scans cannot diagnose laceration of the collecting system; delayed scans (10–30 min) are needed to show extent of contrast leakage

- Shattered kidney (Grade 5): multiple deep lacerations with pieces of kidney held together by vascular scaffolding; some renal parenchyma enhances, other portions are infarcted; large retroperitoneal hematoma usually present; active bleeding from renal artery branches sometimes visible on vascular phase CT

- Total renal infarction (Grade 5): usually caused by dissection/thrombosis of main renal artery; outer renal cortical enhancement ("cortical rim sign") present in only 50% of kidneys acutely, the result of collateral supply from capsular arteries; scans days or weeks later show cortical rim sign more often

- Ureteropelvic junction (UPJ) avulsion: usually in children; hallmark is large amount of extravasated contrast on delayed scans

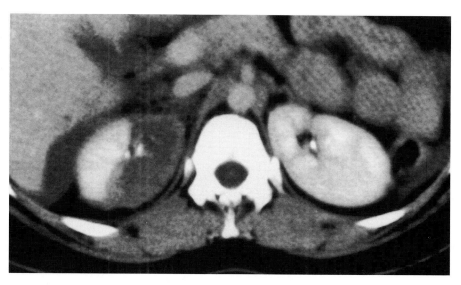

F I G U R E   5 7   Focal right renal infarction, subacute. CT shows geographic region of parenchymal nonperfusion and cortical rim sign.

Renal Injuries: Imaging *(Continued)*

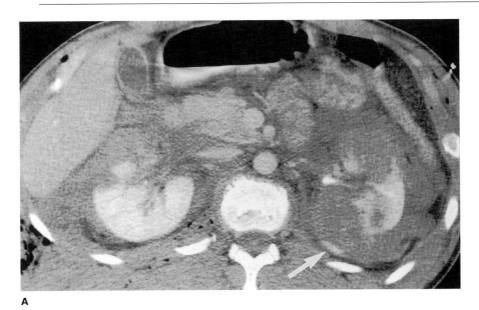

A

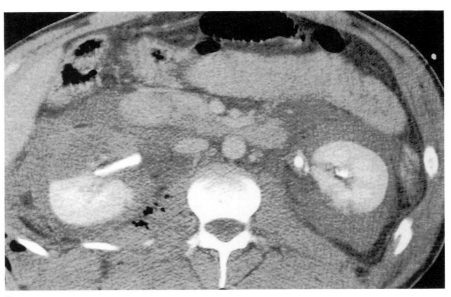

B

F I G U R E   5 8   Bilateral major renal injuries. **(A)** CT shows Grade 3 laceration of right kidney with perinephric hematoma. Left kidney is shattered (Grade 5 injury) with large perinephric hematoma and contrast extravasation posteriorly *(arrow)*. Retroperitoneal gas bubbles are from extensive pulmonary barotrauma. **(B)** More caudal CT slice shows extravasated contrast material adjacent to left ureter, and less severe laceration of the parenchyma at this level. There is an acute infarct in the anterior half of the right kidney, with no cortical rim sign.

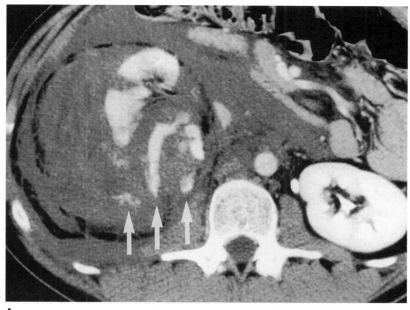

A

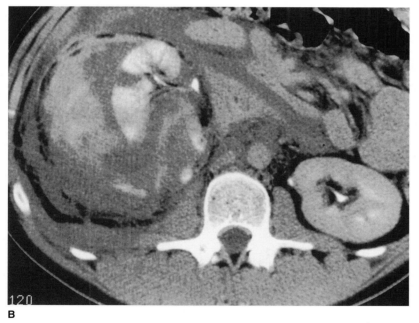

B

F I G U R E 5 9   Shattered right kidney (Grade 5 injury) with active bleeding. **(A)** Vascular phase CT shows enhancing fractured parenchyma, large perinephric, pararenal, and central retroperitoneal hemorrhage, and several sites of extravasation of contrast material *(arrows)* from lacerated blood vessels. The vena cava is compressed by the hematoma. **(B)** Delayed CT scan at 8 minutes, same level as in **(A).** Extravasated contrast has now mixed with hematoma in the perinephric and central retroperitoneal spaces. Excreted contrast opacifies portions of the right collecting system and proximal ureter.

Suggested Reading

Husmann DA, Gilling PJ, Perry MO, Morris JS, Boone TB. Major renal lacerations with a devitalized fragment following blunt abdominal trauma: A comparison between nonoperative (expectant) versus surgical management. *J Urol.* 1993;150:1774-1777.

Renal Injuries: Clinical Management Issues

KEY FACTS

- Vascular pedicle injury and UPJ avulsion usually warrant urgent surgery. When the contralateral kidney is normal, whether or not to attempt revascularization of a kidney with main renal artery dissection/thrombosis is controversial. For other renal injuries, the patient's clinical course is used to determine the need for surgery. Even shattered kidneys sometimes can be managed nonoperatively.

- CT scanning is not reliable in predicting which patients with severe renal injury will require surgery. Large perinephric hematoma (>6 cm), nonresolving or expanding hematoma, and large regions of devitalized parenchyma are associated with a greater likelihood of eventual nephrectomy.

- Reasons for failure of nonsurgical management include: sepsis, coexistent bowel or pancreas injury, failed angio-embolization, delayed diagnosis of ureteral injury, persistent urine leak, urinoma, and refractory hypertension.

- "Page" kidney: chronic subcapsular hematoma causing decreased renal perfusion and increased renin production leading to refractory hypertension.

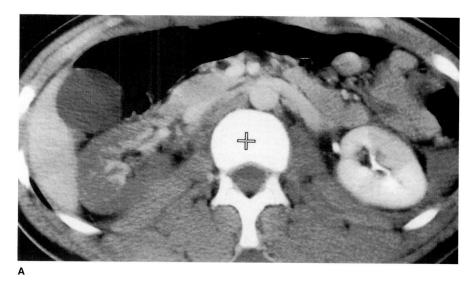

A

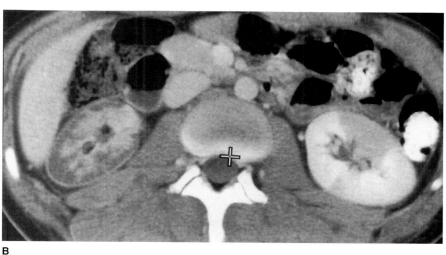

B

F I G U R E 6 0   Traumatic occlusion of right renal artery causing total infarction. **(A)** Contrast enhanced CT scan within hours of injury shows absent parenchymal enhancement except for backflow of contrast laden blood from vena cava into central renal veins. There is no cortical rim sign. Wedge-shaped region of diminished nephrogram in left kidney represents contusion or parenchymal ischemia. **(B)** Repeat scan at 1 week shows well-developed cortical rim sign in right kidney reflecting capsular arterial supply. Central parenchymal enhancement reflects peripelvic collateral blood supply. No change in left kidney region of ischemia or contusion.

Suggested Reading

Lupetin AR, Mainwaring BL, Daffner RH. CT diagnosis of renal artery injury caused by blunt abdominal trauma. *AJR* 1989; 153:1065–1068.

Malmed AS, Love L, Jeffrey RB. Medullary CT enhancement in acute renal artery occlusion. *J Comput Assist Tomogr*. 1992;16:107–109.

Renal Laceration with Urinary Extravasation

KEY FACTS

- Evidence of injury to the collecting system should be sought whenever a deep renal laceration is present. Extravasation of contrast-laden urine may not be visible on the initial CT scan, especially on helical scans performed in the vascular phase. Delayed CT scanning through the kidneys (at least 10 minutes after contrast injection) may be used to show extravasation of opacified urine.

- If the injured kidney does not excrete contrast (e.g., because of total infarction), collecting system or ureteral injury cannot be diagnosed on CT or IVU.

- With renal injury accompanied by perinephric fluid, or with penetrating injury to the retroperitoneum, it is mandatory to visualize the opacified ureter to exclude ureteral injury. If the kidney is excreting contrast, failure to demonstrate the opacified ureter is presumptive evidence of ureteral laceration or avulsion.

- Extravasation of urine from a lacerated kidney is not a surgical emergency. The majority of renal lacerations that extend into the collecting system and cause extravasation can be managed without surgery. Collecting system tears usually heal provided that the path of least resistance for urine is down the ureter.

- Obstruction of the ureter by blood clot may cause absence of ureteral visualization on CT or IVU and promote urine extravasation through a deep parenchymal laceration. Retrograde ureteropyelography must be done to assess the integrity of the UPJ and ureter.

- Potential complications of nonsurgical management of renal laceration with extravasation:

  - Urinoma: A persistent urine leak with an enlarging urinoma requires either ureteral stenting or surgical repair

  - Infection of an injured kidney or urinoma is likely to occur in patients with immunocompromise, bowel injury, or sepsis

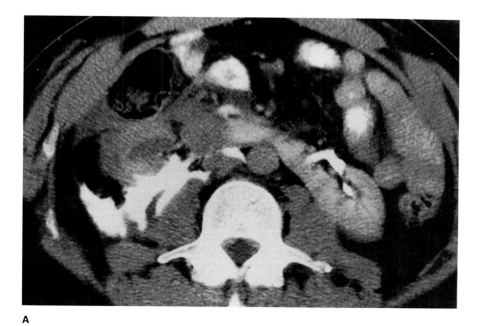

A

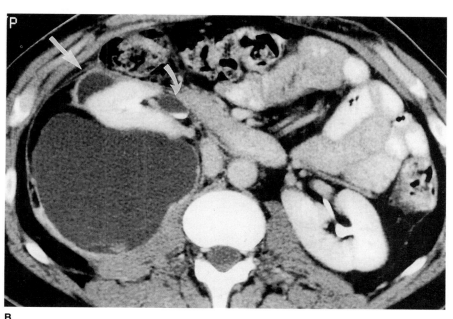

B

F I G U R E   6 1   Horseshoe kidney with Grade 4 laceration and urinoma. **(A)** Contrast enhanced CT scan at level of isthmus. Left side of isthmus is poorly enhanced at site of laceration. Highly concentrated contrast material leaks from the collecting system into the posterior perinephric space. Retrograde ureterogram demonstrated an intact ureter, so patient was managed nonoperatively. **(B)** One month later, CT shows a large posterior fluid collection and a small subcapsular collection anterolaterally *(straight arrow)*. The left renal pelvis is dilated and contains a urine-contrast level *(curved arrow),* suggesting partial obstruction. *(continued)*

Renal Laceration with Urinary Extravasation
(Continued)

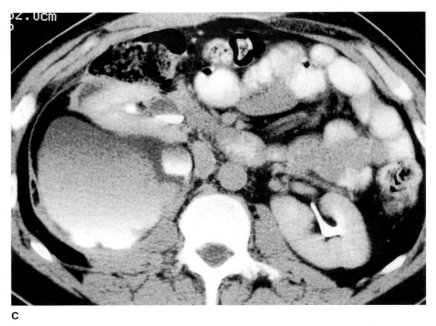

c

F I G U R E   6 1 **(CONTINUED)**   **(C)** CT scan 20 minutes after **(B).** Contrast opacifies the large posterior urinoma. The smaller anterior collection is a subcapsular hematoma. Percutaneous drainage of the urinoma and placement of a ureteral stent allowed the laceration of the pyelocalyceal system to heal.

Suggested Reading
Pollack, HM, Wein AJ. Imaging of renal trauma. *Radiology.* 1989; 172:297–308.

Ureteral Injuries

KEY FACTS

- Most noniatrogenic ureteral injuries are from penetrating trauma and are often associated with injuries to solid organs, major blood vessels, and bowel.

- Ureteral injuries from blunt trauma are most common at the UPJ, followed in frequency by the mid and lower ureter. UPJ disruption may be partial or complete, and is commonly associated with ipsilateral renal parenchymal and/or renal vein laceration. CT is the most accurate examination for detecting ureteral laceration. The "one shot IVU" is reserved for patients who are being taken to surgery straight away. Always inject at least 45 grams of iodine for urgent IVU.

- CT findings of UPJ or proximal ureteric injury:
  - Large fluid collection, predominantly in the postero-medial perinephric space; high attenuation blood and low attenuation urine may be intermixed
  - Nonopacified ureter below site of injury
  - Renal parenchyma may be intact

- Caveats:
  - The distal ureter can still opacify if the proximal laceration is incomplete
  - Renal and proximal ureteral injuries commonly coexist; if major renal parenchymal injury results in absent contrast excretion, a coexistent ureteral laceration will likely be missed

- Vascular phase helical CT cannot demonstrate a urine leak because the kidney will not have excreted contrast so soon after injection. Delayed images (10–20 min) will demonstrate most small or slow leaks; large amounts of extravasated contrast can obscure the source of a leak.

- Even today, most ureteral injuries are not diagnosed before surgery.

Ureteral Injuries (Continued)

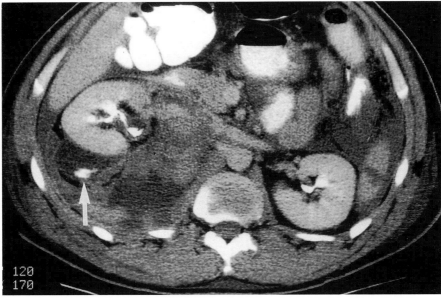

A

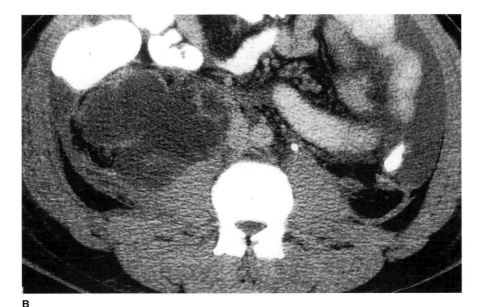

B

F I G U R E   6 2   Proximal ureteral transection from blunt trauma. Value of delayed CT images. **(A)** Contrast enhanced CT shows large mixed attenuation fluid collection medial and posterior to right kidney. Extravasated contrast material is visible near the UPJ, and a small amount pools posteriorly *(arrow)*. **(B)** CT scan in lower lumbar region shows contrast in normal left ureter but no sign of right ureter. The large right retroperitoneal fluid collection contains no contrast at this time. Absent opacification of the ureter, when the kidney is excreting contrast, is presumptive evidence of ureteral transection.

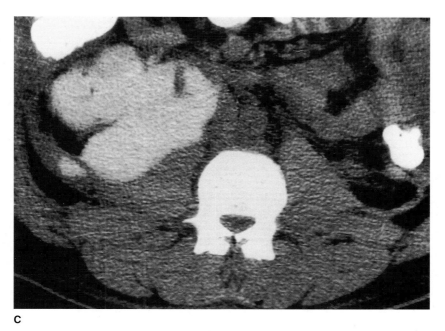

C

F I G U R E   6 2   **(C)** Delayed CT at 7 hours, same level as in **(B).** Contrast material now opacifies the entire urinoma.

Suggested Reading

Kenney PJ, Panicek DM, Witanowski LS. Computed tomography of ureteral disruption. *J Comput Assist Tomogr* 1987;11:480–484.

Kotkin L, Brock JW. Isolated ureteral injury caused by blunt trauma. *Urology* 1996;47: 111–113.

Lang EK. Ureteral injuries. Chapter 52. In: Pollack HM, ed. *Clinical Urography: An Atlas and Textbook of Urological Imaging.* Philadelphia: WB Saunders; 1990:1495–1504.

Bladder Injuries: Extraperitoneal Rupture

KEY FACTS

- Extraperitoneal (EP) bladder rupture accounts for 70-80% of all bladder ruptures from blunt trauma.
- Causes:
  - Blunt trauma: pelvic fracture fragment lacerates bladder; or, shear injury related to disruption of urogenital diaphragm and/or pubovesical fascia
  - Penetrating injury
- Isolated EP bladder rupture can be managed non-operatively with Foley catheter drainage if the laceration is small and the urethra is intact. However, if orthopedic surgery is done to repair pelvic fractures, bladder laceration should be repaired intraoperatively to keep urine away from the surgical site.
- Urine may extravasate into:
  - The perivesical space
  - The anterior prevesical (Retzius) space, sometimes extending cephalad to the umbilicus, and laterally and posteriorly to the retrorectal presacral spaces. The prevesical space is a very large potential space
  - The anterior abdominal fascial layers, including the sheaths of the rectus abdominus muscles
  - The femoral or inguinal canal
  - The scrotum
- Diagnosis of bladder rupture can be made by either radiographic or CT cystography. If a patient needs CT to evaluate abdominal or pelvic bony trauma, CT cystograph should be done at the same time to eliminate extra transfers of the patient.

- Findings on radiographic cystography:
  - Flame-shaped perivesical accumulations of contrast; can dissect along fascial planes of anterior abdominal wall, scrotum, or proximal thigh; on A-P films, cephalad migration of extravasated EP contrast may be mistaken for IP contrast

- Clearcut EP rupture: contrast dissects lateral to bladder and/or into prevesical space; may extend into anterior abdominal wall, scrotum, proximal thigh, or behind rectum.

- Potentially confusing picture: contrast accumulates above and anterior to bladder; large EP extravasation may elevate and compress the peritoneal cavity making it difficult to tell EP from IP contrast; typically, EP contrast will migrate along the anterior abdominal wall and point toward the midline at the umbilicus, in the superior extension of the anterior prevesical space.

- IP contrast tends to move away from midline, toward the paracolic gutters and around bowel loops.

- Combined EP and IP rupture accounts for 5% of bladder ruptures: features of both types of bladder rupture may be demonstrated on cystography, but if one component dominates the picture, the other component can be missed. To better the chance of demonstrating a combined rupture on CT or standard cystography, contrast should be instilled to a bladder pressure of 40 cm H_2O or a volume of 500 ml, whichever comes first, before making the final images.

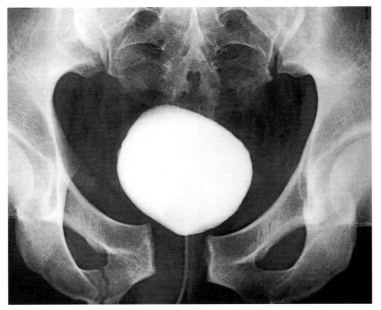

A

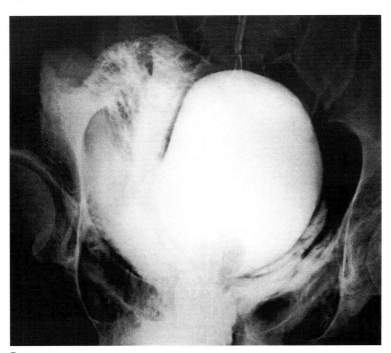

B

F I G U R E   6 3   Extraperitoneal bladder rupture. Importance of adequate bladder distension to avoid falsely negative exam. **(A)** Cystogram with 100 ml of contrast material shows no extravasation. Note pubic and sacroiliac joint diastasis and right inferior pubic ramus fracture. **(B)** With additional contrast material (400 ml) there is extensive extravasation of contrast material into the perivesical tissues and anterior abdominal wall to the right and below the bladder. None of the extrvasated contrast is intraperitoneal.

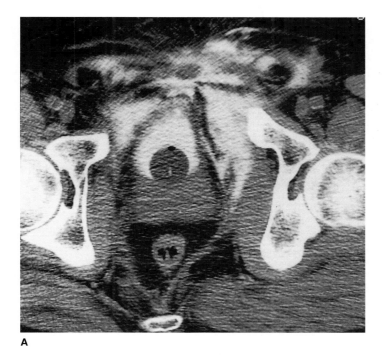

A

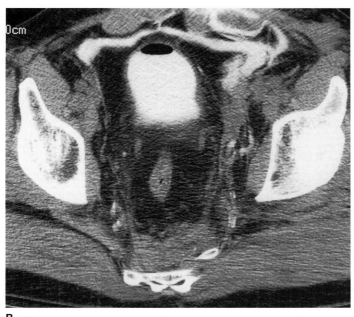

B

F I G U R E   6 4   Extraperitoneal rupture of bladder base. **(A)** CT cystogram, scan near bladder base. Contrast material extravasates extraperitoneally into paravesical spaces, lateral and anterior to bladder. Contrast also enters anterior abdominal wall fascial planes. **(B)** CT cystogram, scan cephalad to that in **(A)**. No hematoma or contrast in the perivesical extraperitoneal fat. Contrast opacifies anterior prevesical space (of Retzius) and extends around right rectus abdominus muscle.

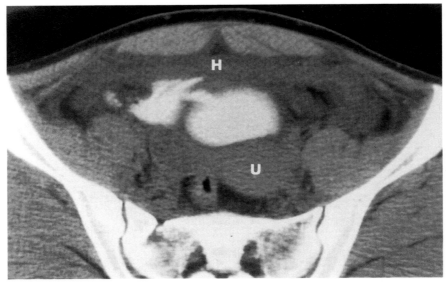

A

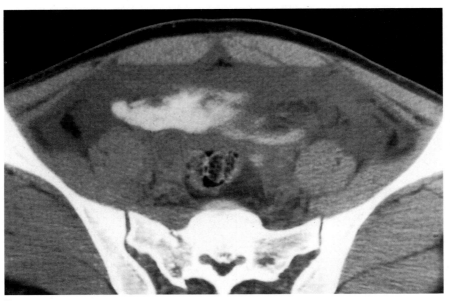

B

FIGURE 65   Extraperitoneal rupture near bladder dome causing potential confusion with intraperitoneal rupture. **(A)** CT cystogram shows contrast extravasation from right side of bladder into perivesical space. There is extensive anterior extraperitoneal hematoma (H). No contrast enters the vesicouterine recess. U = uterus. **(B)** CT cystogram, cephalad to **(A)**. Extravasated contrast mixes with extraperitoneal hematoma anteriorly. No contrast in paracolic gutters or around bowel loops. Exploration confirmed that laceration was entirely extraperitoneal.

Suggested Reading

Corriere JN Jr, Sandler CM. Mechanisms of injury, patterns of extravasation and management of extraperitoneal bladder rupture due to blunt trauma. *J Urol* 1988;139:43–44.

Sandler CM. Bladder trauma. Chapter 53. In: Pollack HM, ed. *Clinical Urography: An Atlas and Textbook of Urological Imaging.* Philadelphia: WB Saunders; 1990:1505–1521.

Bladder Injuries: Intraperitoneal Rupture

KEY FACTS

- Intraperitoneal (IP) rupture accounts for 20% to 30% of bladder ruptures.
- Causes:
  - Blunt lower abdominal or pelvic trauma in a patient with a distended bladder (classic story: automobile accident with intoxicated occupant)
  - Penetrating trauma that lacerates the portion of bladder covered by parietal peritoneum
- IP bladder rupture requires prompt surgical repair.
- Findings on standard and CT cystography:
  - Obvious IP rupture: cystographic contrast collects in the dependent vesicorectal or vesicouterine peritoneal recesses. Larger extravasations cause contrast to flow into the lateral paracolic gutters, around loops of bowel, and under the surface of the liver
- Potentially confusing picture: contrast accumulates cephalad and anterior to bladder; in the absence of contrast material around bowel loops or in the paracolic gutter, this usually represents EP rupture.

Bladder Injuries: Intraperitoneal Rupture
(Continued)

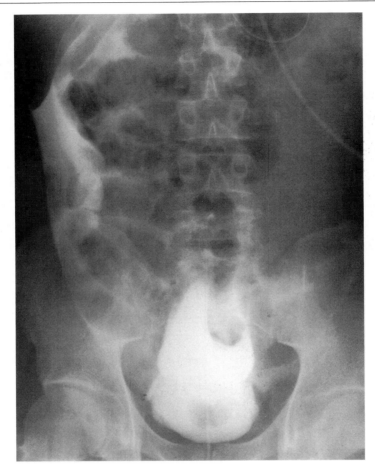

F I G U R E   6 6   Intraperitoneal bladder rupture on standard cystogram. Contrast opacifies vesicorectal pouch, lateral paracolic gutter, Morrison's space, and outlines tip of liver.

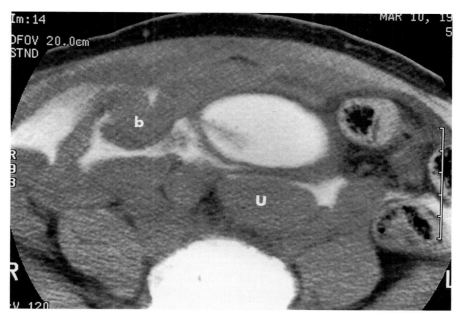

FIGURE 67   Intraperitoneal bladder rupture on CT cystogram. Scan near bladder dome shows laceration of the right side of bladder. Extravasated contrast outlines vesicouterine recess (U = uterus), bowel loop, (B), and both paracolic gutters.

Suggested Reading

Lis LE, Cohen AJ. CT cystography in the evaluation of bladder trauma. *J Comput Assist Tomogr* 1990;14:386–389.

Urethral Injuries

KEY FACTS

- Most urethral injuries occur in men.

- Anatomy: The urethra is divided by the urogenital diaphragm (UGD) into anterior (penile and bulbous) and posterior (membranous and prostatic) portions. The membranous urethra is contained within the UGD and is very short.

- Location and mechanism:
  - Posterior urethra: over 95% are associated with pelvic fractures; 5% to 10% of patients with pelvic fractures have urethral laceration; two-thirds of men with pubic diastatic fracture sustain urethral injury
  - Anterior urethra: straddle injuries to bulbous urethra; iatrogenic (e.g., instrumentation); foreign body

- Clinical signs: inability to void, hematuria, blood at the external meatus, and "high riding" prostate on digital rectal exam. Blood at meatus present in only 50% of patients with urethral trauma.

- Retrograde urethrography (RUG): the examination of choice to evaluate patients with suspected urethral trauma. Brodny clamp, Foley catheter with a small balloon inflated in fossa navicularis, or 8F straight catheter with penile clamp, are acceptable methods (see Protocol Section). "Blind" catheterization can convert a partial urethral tear to a complete disruption.

- Concomitant bladder injury: found in 10% to 20% of men with pelvic fracture and urethral laceration.

- Classification of posterior urethral injuries:
  I. Posterior urethra stretched but not lacerated; hematoma collects in prostatic fossa, displacing bladder base superiorly.
  II. Urethra disrupted at membranoprostatic junction *above* urogenital diaphragm. During RUG, contrast dissects mainly into EP pelvic spaces above the UGD.
  III. Disruption of membranous urethra with extension into proximal bulbous urethra; UGD disrupted; contrast extravasation typically extends above and below UGD.

- Long-term complications of urethral injury in males are stricture, incontinence, and impotence.

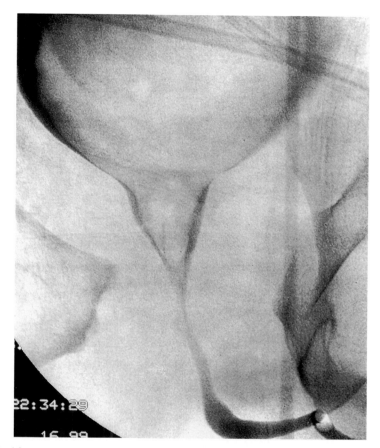

FIGURE 68 Type 1 urethral (stretch) injury. RUG immediately after pelvic arteriography. Marked diastasis of pubic symphysis, elevation of bladder, and elongation of posterior urethra without contrast extravasation. Large intravesical blood clot forms a cast of the widened bladder neck and proximal prostatic urethra.

Urethral Injuries *(Continued)*

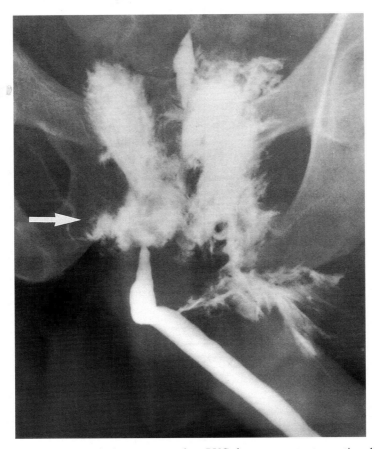

F I G U R E   6 9   Type 2 urethral rupture, complete. RUG shows contrast extravasation above the urogenital diaphragm *(arrow)*. Contrast that extends below the left ischial tuberosity is in the low anterior abdominal wall and thigh. The penile and bulbar urethra are normal.

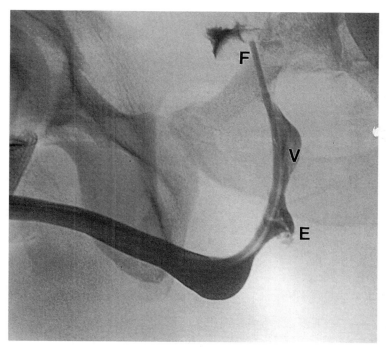

FIGURE 70   Type 3 urethral rupture, partial. Pericatheter RUG shows small extravasation (E) at urogenital diaphragm. Proximal bulbar urethra is narrowed by extrinsic hematoma. Veru montanum (V), Foley catheter balloon (F).

Suggested Reading

Sandler CM, McCallum RW. Injuries of the urethra. Chapter 54. In: Pollack HM, ed. *Clinical Urography: An Atlas and Textbook of Urological Imaging.* Philadelphia: WB Saunders; 1990:1522–1534.

Anterior Urethral Laceration

KEY FACTS

- The most common traumatic injury to the anterior urethra is a partial tear of the bulbous urethra caused by a "straddle" mechanism.

- RUG shows extravasation of contrast into the corpus spongiosum at the site of injury, but the entire anterior urethra is usually opacified; complete rupture is much less common and results in nonvisualization of the urethra proximal to the disruption.

- If Buck's fascia is torn, urine and contrast can dissect into the scrotum and superficial tissues of the abdominal wall.

- Female urethral laceration: due to the short length of the female urethra, injury is less common than in men; diagnosis is usually by direct inspection or VCUG. Retrograde urethrography is technically difficult.

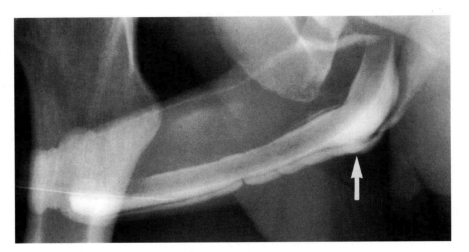

FIGURE 71   Straddle injury to bulbar urethra. Pericatheter RUG shows extravasation of contrast into corpus spongiosum with visualization of dorsal vein. Small laceration in deep bulb *(arrow)*.

Suggested Reading

Sandler CM, Corriere, JN. Urethrography in the diagnosis of acute urethral injuries. *Urol Clin North Am.* 1989;16(2):283–289.

Trauma to the Gravid Uterus

KEY FACTS

- Overall, maternal mortality is the most common cause of fetal demise. In cases where the mother survives her injuries, placental abruption is the most frequent cause of fetal demise.

- Significant placental-fetal injury can occur even in the setting of minor maternal trauma.

- Ultrasound (US) establishes fetal viability and age and helps exclude premature rupture of membranes. Placental abruption may be seen on US, but the sensitivity is as low as 40%. Cardiotocographic (fetal heart and uterine) monitoring are required to confirm fetal well-being and exclude preterm labor and placental abruption.

- Maternal morbidity and mortality pose a much higher risk to the fetus than radiation exposure. Avoid unnecessary and duplicate studies, but do not withhold diagnostic studies necessary for adequate evaluation of maternal injuries.

- Traumatic injury to the fetus itself is uncommon. It occurs in the third trimester because of the decreased amniotic fluid to fetal volume ratio and lower position of the fetal head. Fetal skull fractures and intracranial injuries, associated with maternal pelvic fractures, are typical.

- Uterine rupture is rare; fetal mortality nears 100%.

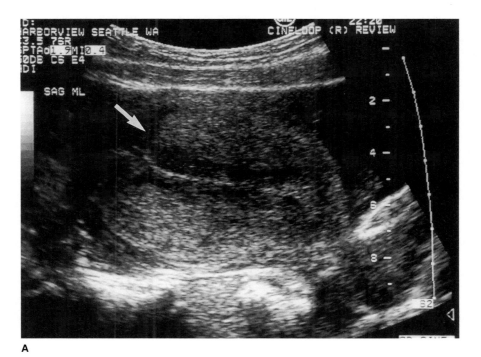

A

FIGURE 72   Uterine rupture on transabdominal US. This woman sustained blunt abdominal trauma in an MVA during the second trimester of her pregnancy. **(A)** Sagittal section through the uterus shows discontinuity of the normal myometrium *(arrow)* indicating the site of uterine rupture. *(continued)*

Trauma to the Gravid Uterus (Continued)

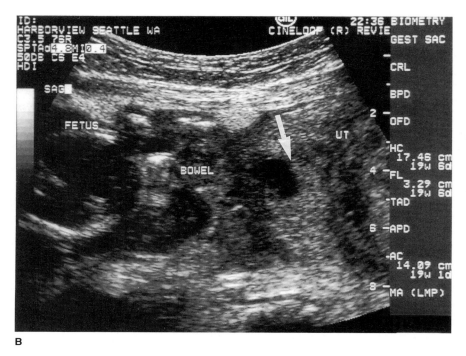

B

F I G U R E   7 2 (CONTINUED)   **(B)** Sagittal section at the maternal mid-abdomen confirms that the 19-week fetus has been ejected from the uterus. The fetal head (FETUS) can be seen in the maternal peritoneal cavity with maternal small bowel (BOWEL) and extruded placenta *(arrow)* interposed between the fetus and the uterine fundus (UT). (Reprinted with permission from *AJR.* 1995;165:1452).

Suggested Reading

Goldman SM, Wagner, LK. Radiologic management of abdominal trauma in pregnancy. *AJR.* 1996;166:763–767.

Testicular Trauma

KEY FACTS

- The spectrum of scrotal injury from penetrating and blunt trauma includes scrotal wall hematoma, hematocele (blood in the tunica vaginalis), and testicular contusion, hematoma, and rupture. Approximately 20% of patients presenting with scrotal trauma will have testicular rupture.

- Urgent surgical treatment of testicular rupture maximizes the probability of salvaging the testis. The presence of scrotal bleeding and swelling hinders the clinical distinction between testicular rupture and less severe scrotal injury.

- Specific ultrasound findings for testicular rupture include:
  - Disruption of testicular contours
  - Extrusion of testicular substance
  - Hypoechoic testicular fracture plane (present in less than 20%)

- Not all cases of testicular rupture will present with specific US findings, although virtually all will have sonographic abnormalities. Patients with a completely normal testicular US can be treated conservatively; those patients at risk for rupture with an abnormal, but nonspecific US, may still warrant surgical exploration.

- The US appearance of hematoceles and testicular hematomas varies depending on their age. In general, they will be hypoechoic acutely, relatively hyperechoic as clot formation progresses and become progressively hypoechoic as clot lysis occurs.

- Color and pulse Doppler assessment of the injured testis confirm adequate blood flow in areas compressed by adjacent hematomas. They can also help in surgical planning for the ruptured testis by identifying potentially devitalized areas.

- Testicular tumors can present with hemorrhage following relatively minor trauma. Color and pulse Doppler may distinguish a vascular tumor from an avascular hematoma. An apparent testicular hematoma, without a history of significant trauma, warrants follow-up US to exclude a neoplasm.

Testicular Trauma (Continued)

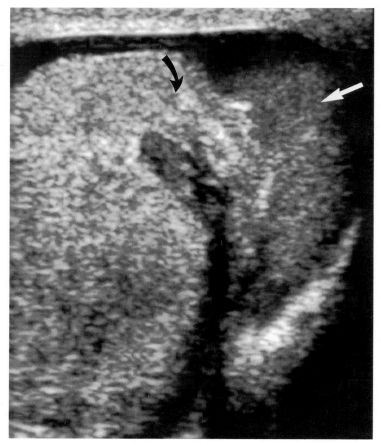

FIGURE 73   Scrotal US from a 34-year-old man with blunt trauma to the right scrotum. Transverse section through the mid-testicle shows extrusion of testicular contents *(curved black arrow)* indicating testicular rupture. There is a hematoma adjacent to the testicle *(white arrow)*.

Suggested Reading
Mulhall JP, Gabram SG, Jacobs LM. Emergency management of blunt testicular trauma. *Acad Emerg Med.* 1995; 2:639–643.

UPPER EXTREMITY

Clavicle Fractures

KEY FACTS

- Clavicle fractures are very common in children, but fortunately heal rapidly and respond well to conservative management.

- Clavicle fractures are classified primarily by location and secondarily by the amount of deformity. The clavicle is a somewhat S-shaped bone with a flat cross-section laterally and a round cross-section medially. This changing cross-section influences the location of fractures. Middle third (group I) fractures account for about 80% of the total, lateral third (group II) account for about 15%, and medial third (group III) only 5%.

- Comminution is not uncommon in all three types. Displacement of the fragments is largely a function of muscle and ligament attachments. Gravity tends to pull the shoulder joint and distal clavicle fragments down, while the muscles tend to hold medial fragments up.

- In distal third fractures (group II), the integrity of the coraco-clavicular ligaments influences the type and severity of displacement. Intact ligaments provide fracture stability.

- Clavicle fractures are usually diagnosed clinically, and the main function of radiographs is to assess the nature and severity of the fracture. Two projections are usually used. One is a straight AP view and the other is AP with the beam directed 45° cephalad.

- Associated subluxations or dislocations of the acromio-clavicular and sternoclavicular joints are often present.

- Clavicle fractures are most commonly isolated injuries. Associated injuries to the lung apex, subclavian vessels, brachial plexus, and first rib are infrequent.

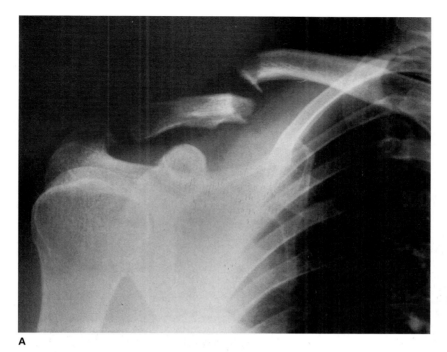

A

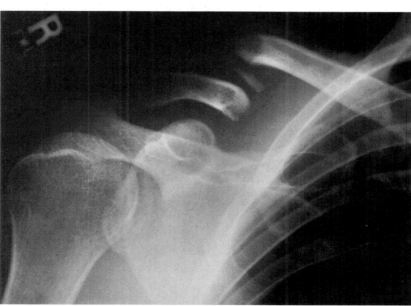

B

FIGURE 1 **(A)** AP and **(B)** up-angled AP views of a comminuted clavicular shaft fracture. Note the upward displacement of the proximal fragment. The distal fragment moves with the scapula, confirming the integrity of the coraco-clavicular ligaments.

Suggested Reading

Rogers LF. In: *Radiology of Skeletal Trauma*. New York: Churchill Livingstone; 1992: 658–662.

Craig EV. In: Rockwood CA, Green DP, Bucholz RW, eds. *Rockwood and Green's Fractures*. Philadelphia: Lippincott; 1991:928–983.

Mayo KA, Swiontkowski MF. In: Hansen ST, Swiontkowski MF. eds. *Orthopaedic Trauma Protocols*. New York: Raven Press; 1993:77–79.

Acromio-Clavicular Joint Dislocation

KEY FACTS

- The acromioclavicular joint is supported by a thin fibrous capsule and by discrete acromioclavicular ligaments situated anteriorly, posteriorly, superiorly, and inferiorly. Further support for this joint is provided by the coracoclavicular ligaments.

- The exact relationship between the acromion and clavicle varies, with orientation of the joint being anywhere from parallel to the glenoid to 50° of obliquity. The clavicle can lie somewhat superior to the acromion, a normal variant that should not be mistaken for traumatic dissociation.

- Acromioclavicular joint injuries are classified into three types, according to the associated ligament injuries:

    - Type I is a simple sprain of the acromioclavicular ligaments (without frank rupture), and radiographically shows no joint displacement

    - Type II has disrupted acromioclavicular ligaments, allowing some displacement of the joint, but the coracoclavicular ligaments are intact, preventing complete dissociation

    - Type III has disruption of both the acromioclavicular and coracoclavicular ligaments with complete dissociation of the scapula and clavicle

  Type I and II injuries are usually managed conservatively. Type III injuries are usually repaired surgically.

- The acromioclavicular joint is best seen on modified AP views of the shoulder with the beam angled 10° to 15° cephalad. The opposite joint should be imaged for comparison, to allow for the large variations in normal anatomy. The radiographs should be obtained with the patient sitting or standing and the arms hanging loosely at the sides. A second similar examination should then be performed, with 10 to 15 pound weights in each hand, to evaluate instability.

- In some Type II injuries, the acromioclavicular displacement can actually decrease with weights as the patient contracts the shoulder muscles in reaction to the load. This still represents joint laxity—any motion with weight bearing should be considered abnormal.

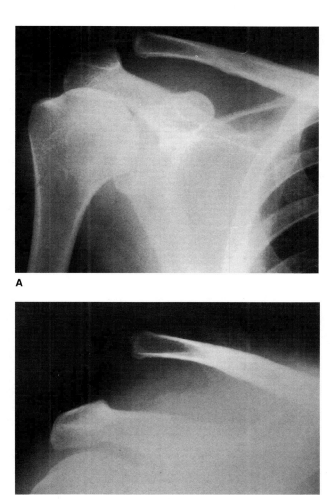

F I G U R E 2   AP radiographs of a type III acromioclavicular joint injury, **(A)** with and **(B)** without weights. Note the wide displacement that occurs with weight bearing, confirming complete disruption of both the acromio-clavicular and coraco-clavicular ligaments. The joint is clearly very unstable.

Suggested Reading

Mayo KA, Swiontkowski MF. In: Hansen ST, Swiontkowski MF. eds. *Orthopaedic Trauma Protocols*. New York: Raven Press; 1993:80–83.

Rockwood CA, Williams GR, Young DC. In: Rockwood CA, Green DP, Bucholz RW. eds. *Rockwood and Green's Fractures*. Philadelphia: Lippincott; 1991:1181–1239.

Shoulder Joint Dislocation

KEY FACTS

- Dislocations of the shoulder joint account for more than half of all major joint dislocations.

- A dislocation is defined as separation between the glenoid fossa and humeral head articular surfaces that will not spontaneously reduce. A subluxation, on the other hand, is defined as symptomatic incomplete separation of the articular surfaces that is transient and reduces spontaneously.

- Shoulder dislocations are classified according to the position of the humeral head, relative to the glenoid labrum. The positions in which the head can reside are anterior, posterior, inferior, and superior.

- Anterior dislocations account for more than 90% of the total and posterior dislocations account for most of the remainder. Inferior dislocations are very uncommon and superior dislocations are rare. The rarest variant is intrathoracic dislocation, with the humeral head protruding through the chest wall.

- In anterior dislocations, the humeral head is displaced not only anteriorly, but also medially and inferiorly; to a subcoracoid position (Figure 3). The resultant deformity is readily visible both clinically and radiographically. Associated fractures of the glenoid margin (Bankart fractures) and humeral head (Hill-Sachs fractures) are common.

- In posterior dislocations, the humeral head lies directly behind the glenoid, usually with minimal medial displacement (Figure 5).

- In inferior dislocations (also known as "luxatio erecta") the humeral head lies directly below the glenoid and the shaft of the humerus is fixed in marked abduction (Figure 4). This deformity is obvious both clinically and radiographically.

- Adequate evaluation requires good quality conventional radiographs (with the same projections as scapular fractures).

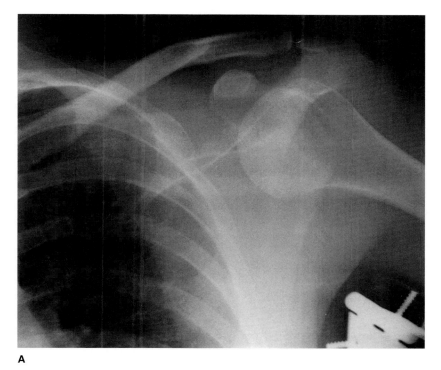

A

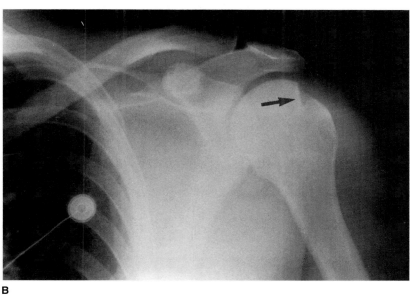

B

F I G U R E   3   Anterior shoulder dislocation. **(A)** AP view following injury shows the humeral head lying anterior and inferior to the glenoid fossa. **(B)** A postreduction AP view shows not only that the dislocation has been reduced but that there is a Hill-Sachs impaction fracture *(black arrow)* on the posterosuperior margin of the humeral head. *(continued)*

Shoulder Joint Dislocation *(Continued)*

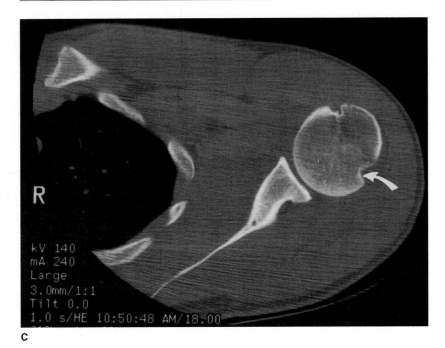

C

F I G U R E 3 (CONTINUED)   **(C)** CT scan shows the Hill-Sachs fracture *(curved white arrow)* even more clearly.

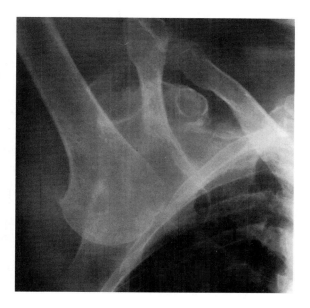

FIGURE 4

Shoulder Dislocation—Luxatio Erecta. A single AP view shows the humeral head lying anteromedial and inferior to the glenoid fossa with the arm fixed in abduction. Incidentally noted is a superior glenoid margin fracture.

Suggested Reading

Mayo KA, Swiontkowski MF. In: Hansen ST, Swiontkowski, MF. eds. *Orthopaedic Trauma Protocols.* New York: Raven Press; 1993:86–87.

Rockwood CA, Thomas SA, Matsen FA. In: Rockwood CA, Green DP, Bucholz RW. eds. *Rockwood and Green's Fractures.* Philadelphia: Lippincott; 1991:1041–1142.

Shoulder Dislocation: Posterior

KEY FACTS

- The subtle deformity in posterior shoulder dislocation can easily be overlooked by the unwary physician, both clinically and radiographically.

- Associated injuries such as humeral neck fractures can occur. Such injuries can draw the attention of the unwary physician away from the less conspicuous dislocation.

- Most reports in the literature list failed diagnosis rates close to 50%. Failure rates this high cannot be justified, since all of these injuries can be diagnosed with adequate radiographs.

- A Grashey (posterior oblique) or Standard AP radiograph combined with a lateral scapular ("Y") view should be considered the minimum evaluation. Axillary views may be difficult to obtain, but do provide useful information about the relative positions of the glenoid fossa and humeral head.

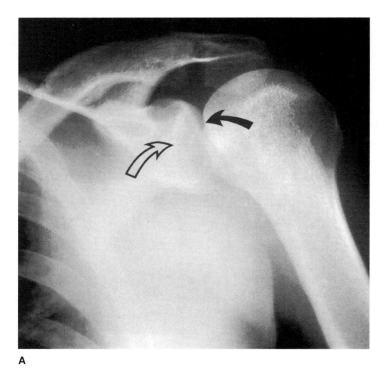

A

F I G U R E   5   **(A)** The AP view of a posteriorly dislocated shoulder shows humeral head *(closed arrow)* separated from glenoid fossa *(open arrow).*

- The important signs on the Grashey and AP views are: overlap of the humeral head and glenoid articular surfaces, imperfect alignment of the humeral head with the glenoid fossa (too high or too low), persistent internal rotation of the humerus on all views, and the presence of the "trough line".

- The "trough line" represents an impaction fracture of the anterior articular surface of the humeral head. It is most commonly seen on AP projections as a curved dense line that parallels the articular margin of the humeral head (Figure 5). These fractures are relatively common associates in posterior dislocations.

- The posterior internally rotated position of the head is readily confirmed by both the "Y" and axillary views.

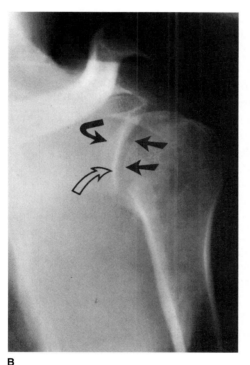

B

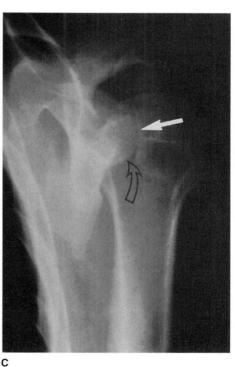

C

F I G U R E   5   **(B)** The Grashey view shows overlap of the humeral head *(curved arrow)* and glenoid fossa *(open arrow)* with a third curved line *(two arrows)* in the humeral head representing the trough line of an impacted articular surface fracture. This fracture is also shown on **(C)** the "Y" view *(white arrow),* impacted onto the margin of the glenoid fossa *(open arrow).*

Suggested Reading

Rogers LF. In: *Radiology of Skeletal Trauma.* New York: Churchill Livingstone; 1992: 732–742.

Rockwood CA, Thomas SA, Matsen FA. In: Rockwood CA, Green DP, Bucholz RW. eds. *Rockwood and Green's Fractures.* Philadelphia: Lippincott; 1991:1041–1142.

Proximal Humeral Fractures

K E Y   F A C T S

- Injuries to the proximal humerus include fractures of the head, neck, and tuberosities. Humeral neck fractures are the most common and typically involve the surgical (rather than the anatomic) neck. Articular and periarticular fractures of the humeral head are usually associated with joint dislocations or subluxations. Isolated tuberosity fractures are the least disabling of these injuries.

- The most widely used classification for surgical neck fractures was developed by Neer. This classification simply counts the number of major displaced fragments and defines the specific parts involved. It does not include non-displaced fractures.

- The major parts included in the Neer classification are the greater and lesser tuberosities, humeral head, and humeral shaft. A displaced fracture can have two, three, or four of these parts.

- The humeral head tends to remain in the glenoid fossa, while the other three fragments are displaced away from it. The direction of displacement of each of these fragments is a function of their muscle attachments.

- The greater tuberosity is pulled superiorly and posteriorly by supraspinatus and infraspinatus, the lesser tuberosity is pulled medially by subscapularis, and the shaft is pulled medially by pectoralis major.

- The presence or absence of articular surface involvement is important. Fractures splitting the humeral head can also occur, either as part of more complex head and neck fractures or as isolated injuries. Humeral head fractures that simply indent the surface of the bone are most commonly the result of dislocations.

- Complications are relatively infrequent in humeral neck fractures but include, avascular necrosis, nonunion, malunion, infection, neurovascular injury, hardware failure, and frozen shoulder.

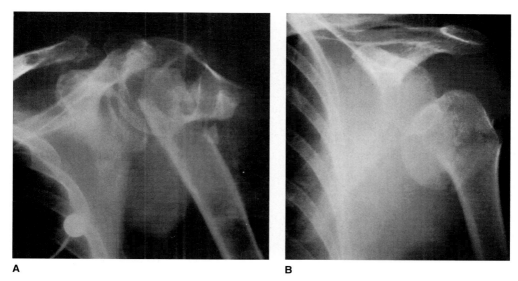

A   B

F I G U R E   6   **(A)** Markedly displaced two part humeral neck fracture with abduction and external rotation of the proximal fragment by the rotator cuff muscles. The shaft is displaced medially by the pectoralis major. **(B)** Minimally displaced impacted humeral neck fracture in another patient, 2 days post-injury. Note how the humeral head has subluxed inferiorly out of the glenoid fossa, secondary to hemarthrosis and muscle weakness. This should not be confused with a shoulder dislocation.

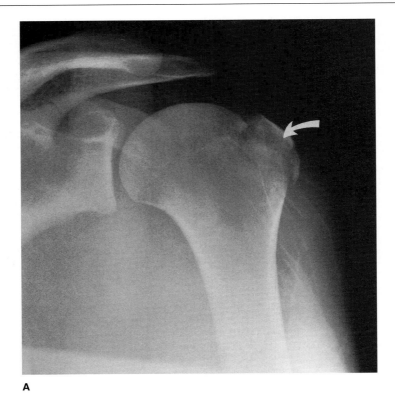

A

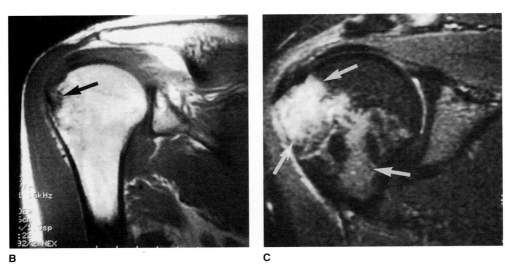

B   **C**

FIGURE 7   **(A)** AP shoulder radiograph, showing comminuted, avulsed, greater tuberosity *(arrow)*. **(B)** T1-weighted and **(C)** STIR images from MRI scan of another patient, showing extensive bone marrow edema *(arrowheads)* around a nondisplaced greater tuberosity fracture. In this patient, the fracture was not visible on shoulder radiographs.

Suggested Reading

Rogers LF. In: *Radiology of Skeletal Trauma*. New York: Churchill Livingstone; 1992: 696–710.

Bigliani LU. In: Rockwood CA, Green DP, Bucholz RW. eds. *Rockwood and Green's Fractures*. Philadelphia: Lippincott; 1991:871–920.

Humeral Shaft Fractures

KEY FACTS

- Humeral shaft fractures are classified by location: Above pectoralis major insertion; below pectoralis major, but above deltoid insertion; below deltoid insertion.

- These fractures are also classified by direction and character of fracture: longitudinal; transverse; oblique; spiral; segmental; comminuted; open; closed.

- The location of the fracture impacts the way in which the fragments are displaced.

- Humeral shaft fractures can be associated with injuries to the brachial vessels.

- These fractures can be associated with injuries to the radial, ulnar, and median nerves. Radial nerve injuries are the commonest.

- The radial nerve is injured in about 10% of cases leading to wrist-drop that can be permanent, if the nerve is transected.

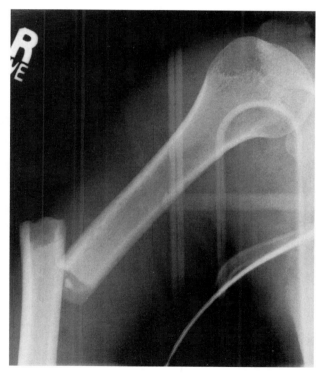

FIGURE 8   This patient sustained a transverse mid-shaft humeral fracture in a motor-vehicle accident. There is greater than 100% displacement with shortening and marked angulation. The shortening has resulted from the forearm extensors and flexors pulling the distal fragment proximally and the angulation has resulted from the abductors of the shoulder pulling the proximal fragment laterally.

Suggested Reading

Rogers LF. In: *Radiology of Skeletal Trauma*. New York: Churchill Livingstone; 1992: 710–716.

Epps CH, Grant RE. In: Rockwood CA, Green DP, Bucholz RW. eds. *Rockwood and Green's Fractures*. Philadelphia: Lippincott; 1991:843–867.

Distal Humeral Fractures

KEY FACTS

- Distal humeral fractures are classified by their relationship to the humeral condyles. Four types are described: supracondylar, intercondylar, condylar, and epicondylar.

- Supracondylar fractures are most the common and are usually seen in children aged 9 to 12 years.

- Supracondylar fractures are due to hyperextension, with posterior angulation and displacement of the condyles.

- Supracondylar fractures are subclassified into three types:
  - Type I. Nondisplaced
  - Type II. Displaced with posterior cortical continuity
  - Type III. Totally displaced

- Intercondylar ("T" and "Y") fractures are subclassified into four types:
  - Type I. Nondisplaced
  - Type II. Displaced
  - Type III. Displaced and rotated
  - Type IV. Displaced, rotated, and comminuted

- Condylar fractures involve the capitellum and trochlea either separately or together.

- Epicondylar fractures occur both medially and laterally.

- Anteroposterior and lateral radiographs of the elbow are usually adequate to evaluate distal humeral fractures.

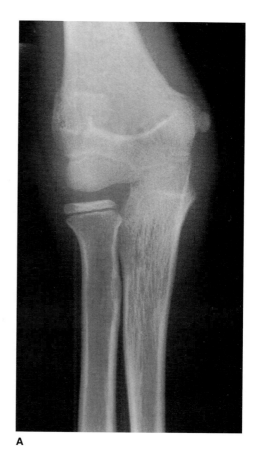

A

FIGURE 9

Type II supracondylar fracture. This 12-year-old boy
fell onto his outstretched hand. **(A)** AP and **(B)** lateral
views of the elbow show a typical supracondylar
fracture. The distal fracture fragment can be seen on
the lateral view to be tilted posteriorly, but it is still
articulating normally with the radius and ulna.

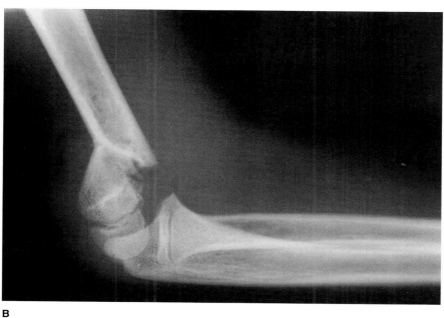

B

Suggested Reading

Rogers LF. In: *Radiology of Skeletal Trauma*. New York: Churchill Livingstone; 1992:
759–772.

Hotchkiss RN, Green DP. In: Rockwood CA, Green DP, Bucholz RW. eds. *Rockwood and
Green's Fractures*. Philadelphia: Lippincott; 1991:739–774.

Humerus: Epicondyle Injury

KEY FACTS

- While direct injury to the epicondyles is possible, most epicondylar fractures are the result of avulsion.
- Medial epicondyle fractures are much more common than lateral and are usually seen in children, prior to physeal closure.
- The medial epicondyle provides the common origin for the forearm flexor muscles and is avulsed when sudden stress is applied to these muscles.
- Medial epicondyle avulsion is also associated with elbow dislocations and the epicondyle can become trapped within the elbow joint, prior to or during reduction.
- The medial epicondyle is usually displaced distally but the displacement is not always obvious radiographically and a comparison view of the opposite elbow is often helpful.
- The lateral epicondyle provides the common origin for the forearm extensors and can be avulsed in a similar fashion to the medial epicondyle. This injury, however, is infrequent.

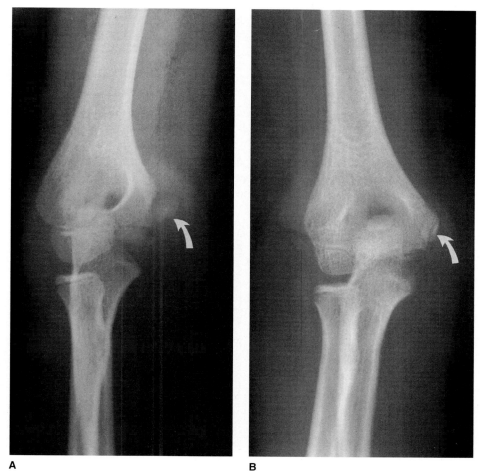

A   B

FIGURE 10   This child has avulsed his right medial humeral epicondyle. **(A)** AP view of the injured elbow with the medial epicondyle *(arrow)* displaced medially. The normal position of the epicondyle *(arrow)* is shown on **(B)** an AP view of the opposite (normal) elbow that was obtained for comparison. The radiograph of the normal elbow has been reversed so that the anatomy of the two sides will match.

Suggested Reading

Rogers LF. In: *Radiology of Skeletal Trauma.* New York: Churchill Livingstone; 1992: 772–784.

Hotchkiss RN, Green DP. In: Rockwood CA, Green DP, Bucholz RW. eds. *Rockwood and Green's Fractures.* Philadelphia: Lippincott; 1991:775–779.

Elbow Dislocation

KEY FACTS

- The elbow joint is very stable and therefore dislocates less frequently than the shoulder joint.

- Elbow dislocations are classifiesd by the position of the ulna relative to the humerus. Most are posterior, but anterior, lateral, medial, and divergent types are possible.

- Associated fractures can occur, affecting the medial humeral epicondyle, the coronoid and olecranon processes of the ulna, the radial head, and the articular surfaces of the elbow joint.

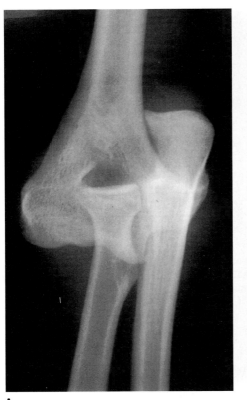 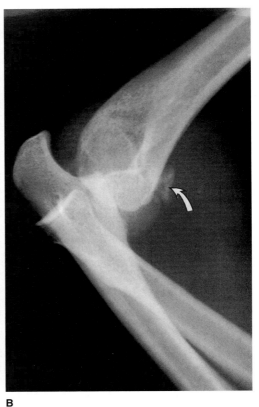

A **B**
FIGURE 11

(A) AP and (B) lateral views of the elbow show complete dislocation, with medial and posterior displacement of the forearm bones. A small bony fragment *(arrows)* has been avulsed from the coronoid process.

- Medial epicondyle and coronoid fractures are the most common associated injuries and have been reported in up to 60% of dislocations.

- Injuries to the brachial vessels, and radial, ulnar, or median nerves are uncommon.

- Typically the radial head and proximal ulna dislocate together.

- Isolated radial head or ulnar dislocations are rare in adults, but are more common in young children.

- As with dislocations in other large joints, the diagnosis is obvious clinically, and the main roles of radiography are to categorize the injury and detect associated fractures. Standard AP and lateral views are usually adequate for these injuries.

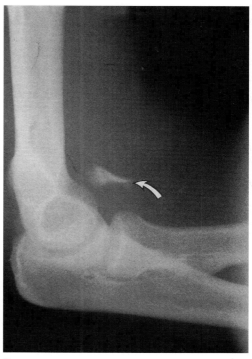

FIGURE 11

The avulsion is more apparent on **(C)** the post-reduction lateral view.

C

Suggested Reading

Rogers LF. In: *Radiology of Skeletal Trauma*. New York: Churchill Livingstone; 1992: 805–811.

Hotchkiss RN, Green DP. In: Rockwood CA, Green DP, Bucholz RW. eds. *Rockwood and Green's Fractures*. Philadelphia: Lippincott; 1991:779–794.

Radial Head Fractures

K E Y F A C T S

- Radial head fractures are intra-articular and usually produce hemarthroses.
- The hemarthrosis can be identified by displacement of the elbow fat pads on lateral radiographs.
- Radial head fractures can be difficult to see on standard AP and lateral radiographs.
- Oblique views and special radial head views may be needed to see nondisplaced and marginal fractures. The radial head view is performed with the elbow bent, the arm and film horizontal, and the central ray directed 45° cephalad.
- Radial head fractures should be suspected in all elbow injuries when there is pain and tenderness laterally with displaced fat pads visible on lateral radiographs.
- Radial head fractures can also be associated with injuries to the interosseous membrane.
- Complete interosseous membrane ruptures will produce acute longitudinal radio-ulnar dissociation (ALRUD), otherwise known as the Essex-Lopresti injury.

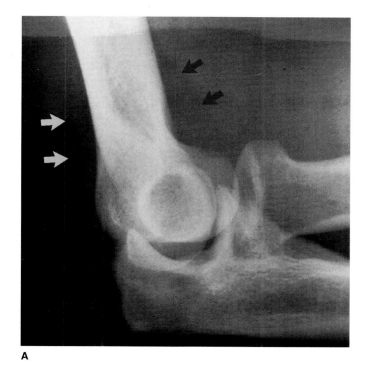

A

B

FIGURE 12   **(A)** The lateral view shows displaced fat pads *(arrows)* indicating a joint effusion. The fracture is not apparent on this view, nor was it seen on the AP projection. **(B)** A radial head view shows the slightly comminuted radial head fracture *(arrows)* well.

Suggested Reading

Rogers LF. In: *Radiology of Skeletal Trauma*. New York: Churchill Livingstone; 1992: 788–799.

Hotchkiss RN, Green DP. In: Rockwood CA, Green DP, Bucholz RW. eds. *Rockwood and Green's Fractures*. Philadelphia: Lippincott; 1991:805–824.

Radius and Ulna Shaft Fractures

KEY FACTS

- The radius and ulna are coupled proximally and distally, by the radio-ulnar joints, forming a fibro-osseous ring. Such rings are stable if fractured in one place but are unstable if fractured in two places.

- A direct blow to a forearm bone can produce a stable single bone fracture. This occurs most commonly in the ulna and is known as the "night-stick" fracture.

- Unstable forearm injuries are usually the result of indirect trauma, most commonly a fall onto the outstretched hand.

- Both-bone forearm fractures are the most common unstable injuries, these occur typically near the mid forearm. Rotational deformity is common with the wrist pronated and the proximal radius supinated.

- A fracture of the proximal ulnar shaft associated with dislocation of the proximal radio-ulnar joint is known as a Monteggia fracture and should be suspected whenever an isolated proximal ulnar fracture is seen.

- A fracture of the distal radial shaft associated with dislocation of the distal radio-ulnar joint is known as a Galleazzi fracture. This injury should be suspected whenever an isolated distal radial shaft fracture is present, particularly if there is displacement, angulation or shortening.

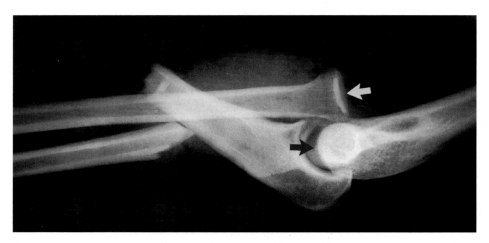

FIGURE 13   Monteggia fracture. A lateral view of the elbow shows a proximal ulnar shaft fracture with marked displacement, angulation, and shortening. Note that the radial head *(white arrow)* is dislocated from its normal articulation with the capitellum *(black arrow)*.

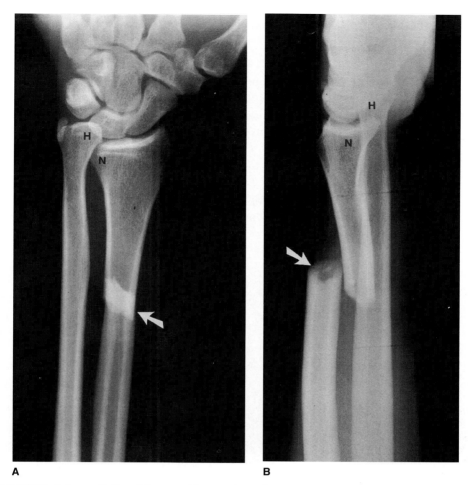

A **B**

FIGURE 14   Galleazzi fracture. **(A)** AP and **(B)** lateral views of the distal forearm show a displaced, angulated, and shortened fracture *(arrows)* of the distal radial shaft. The ulnar head (H) is displaced distally and palmarly, out of its normal articulation (N) with the distal radius.

Suggested Reading

Rogers LF. In: *Radiology of Skeletal Trauma*. New York: Churchill Livingstone; 1992: 811–825.

Anderson LD, Myer FN. In: Rockwood CA, Green DP, Bucholz RW. eds. *Rockwood and Green's Fractures*. Philadelphia: Lippincott; 1991:679–734.

Distal Radius and Ulna Fractures

KEY FACTS

- Distal radius and ulna fracture patterns vary with patient age. These fractures result most commonly from a fall onto the outstretched hand.

- Prepubescent children are most likely to have buckle (torus) fractures of the distal radial metaphysis or greenstick fractures of the distal shafts of both bones (Figure 15).

- Adolescents are most likely to have fractures involving the distal radial physis (Salter-Harris injuries).

- Adults will tend to have complete fractures of the distal radial metadiaphyseal region, often associated with fractures of the ulnar styloid

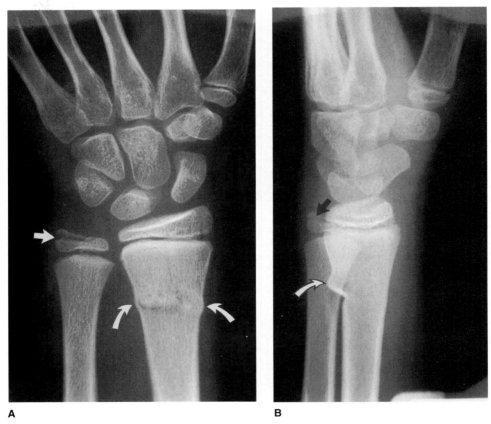

A   **B**

FIGURE 15   Torus fracture. **(A)** AP and **(B)** lateral views of a 9-year-old girl's wrist show a fracture *(curved arrows)* through the distal radius. The buckling nature of the injury is best appreciated on the lateral view. There is also a fracture through the ulnar styloid in this patient *(straight arrows).*

process. These fractures are most common in older, osteoporotic individuals.

- Distal radial fractures in adults with dorsal angulation and/or displacement of the distal fragment are known as Colles fractures (Figure 16).

- When the distal radial fracture fragment is angulated and/or displaced palmarly, it is called a Smith's fracture.

- Fracture-dislocations of the radiocarpal joint (involving the distal radius) are known as a Barton's fractures. Barton's fractures are classified as either dorsal or palmar, depending on the direction of displacement of the carpus.

- An anteriorly displaced, intra-articular, Smith's fracture and a palmar Barton's fracture are the same injury (Figure 17).

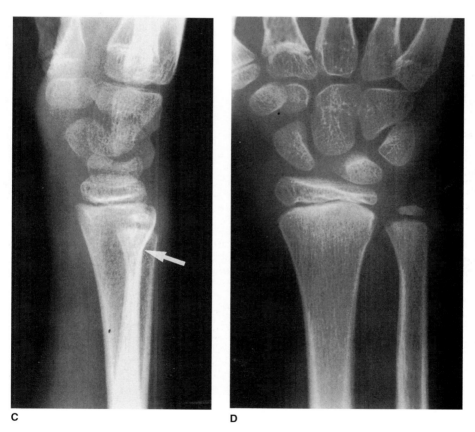

C   D

FIGURE 15   Torus fractures can be very subtle, as demonstrated by **(C)** the lateral view of a 7-year-old boy's wrist where the fracture *(arrow)* is seen simply as a sudden change in angulation of the distal radius. In this second patient, the fracture is not visible on **(D)** the AP view. Follow-up films showed clear evidence of healing with a line of sclerosis across the distal radius.

Distal Radius and Ulna Fractures (Continued)

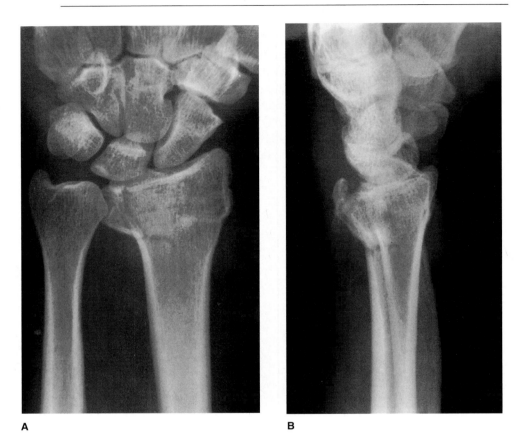

A   **B**

FIGURE 16   Colles fracture. This elderly woman fell onto her outstretched hand, sustaining a transverse fracture through the metadiaphyseal region of her distal radius. **(A)** AP and **(B)** lateral views of the wrist show that the fracture is slightly comminuted and extends into the distal radial articular surface. The lateral view also shows dorsal tilting of the distal fracture fragment.

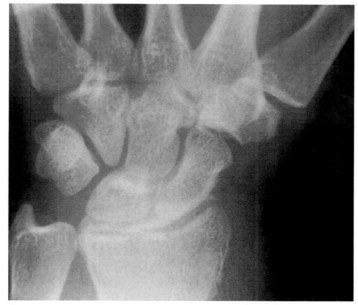

A

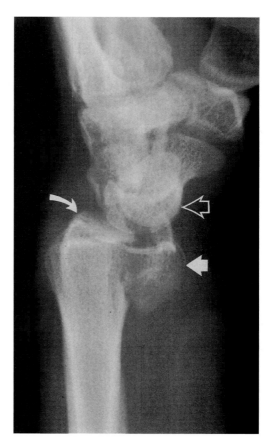

B

FIGURE 17

Anterior (palmar) Barton's fracture. **(A)** AP and **(B)** lateral views of an adult wrist show fracture dislocation of the radiocarpal joint. On the lateral view, we can see that the palmar fracture fragment *(closed broad arrow)* still articulates with the proximal carpal row *(open broad arrow),* while the remainder of the distal radius *(curved arrow)* lies dorsal to the carpus.

Suggested Reading

Rogers LF. In: *Radiology of Skeletal Trauma*. New York: Churchill Livingstone; 1992: 837–870.

Cooney WP, Linscheid RL, Dobyns JH. In: Rockwood CA, Green DP, Bucholz RW. eds. *Rockwood and Green's Fractures*. Philadelphia: Lippincott; 1991:585–601.

Carpal Fractures

K E Y   F A C T S

- The scaphoid is the commonest carpal bone fractured. These fractures are seen most frequently in young adults and usually result from a fall on the outstretched hand.

- Most scaphoid fractures occur through the midportion (waist) of the bone (Figure 18).

- The blood supply to the proximal pole of the scaphoid can be compromised by waist fractures and is always compromised by proximal pole fractures.

- Delayed union is common when there is vascular compromise and can lead to nonunion or to ischemic necrosis.

- Distal pole and tubercle fractures (Figure 19) are not subject to vascular compromise and usually heal well.

- Most scaphoid fractures are minimally displaced. When there is marked displacement, associated ligament injuries and carpal dislocations should be suspected.

- The second most common carpal bone to fracture is the triquetrum (Figure 20). These fractures usually take the form of dorsal chips. They represent ligament avulsions and generally have a good prognosis.

- A complete four-view series of PA, oblique, lateral, and scaphoid views is essential to adequately evaluate the carpus (Figures 18, 19, 20). Each one of the views will show injuries that are difficult to see on the other three. The scaphoid view is taken in full ulnar deviation with the central ray angulated 20° cephalad.

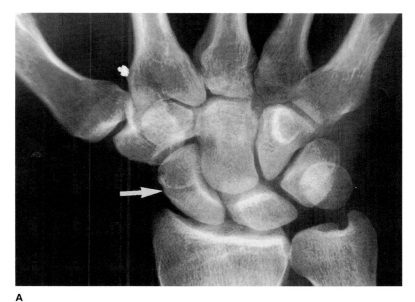

F I G U R E   1 8   Scaphoid waist fracture. The fracture *(arrow)* is difficult to see on **(A)** the standard PA view, but it is clearly visible on **(B)** the scaphoid view. This fracture was not visible on either the oblique or lateral views.

Carpal Fractures (Continued)

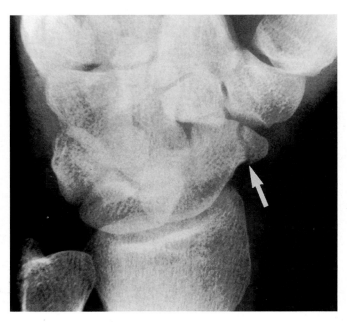

FIGURE 19   Scaphoid tubercle fracture. While this oblique view clearly shows the fracture *(arrow),* it could not be found on the PA view.

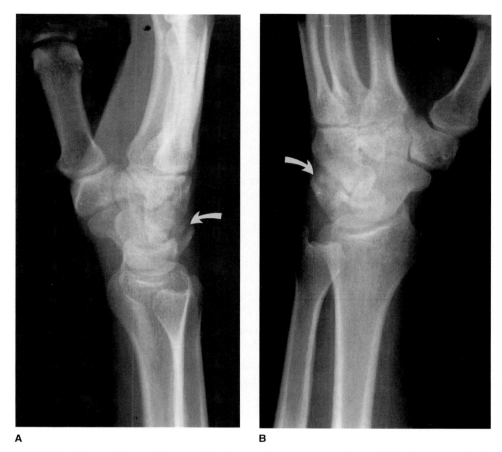

A   **B**

F I G U R E   2 0   Triquetral fracture. This fracture *(arrows)* was visible on **(A)** the lateral and **(B)** the oblique views, but was not shown by the other two views of the wrist.

Suggested Reading

Yin Y, Mann FA, Gilula LA. In: Gilula LA, Yin Y. eds. *Imaging of the Wrist and Hand.* Philadelphia: WB Saunders; 1996:93–157.

Rogers LF. In: *Radiology of Skeletal Trauma.* New York: Churchill Livingstone; 1992: 870–910.

Carpal Dislocations

KEY FACTS

- The majority of carpal dislocations occur around the lunate, through the midcarpal joint.

- There is a zone of vulnerability that extends in an arc-like fashion across the carpus. It begins laterally at the radial styloid and expands across the scaphoid bone, through the proximal capitate and midcarpal joint, across the luno-triquetral joint, and onto the ulnar styloid process.

- These dislocations are classified as perilunate if the lunate continues to articulate with the radius. They are called lunate dislocations when the lunate is dislocated out of its radial articulation. An intermediate state has been labeled as a midcarpal dislocation by some experts.

- The most common variant of the lunate/perilunate series is the trans-scaphoid-perilunate dislocation (Figure 21). As its name implies, this midcarpal joint disruption includes a scaphoid waist fracture and a perilunate dislocation. It also frequently includes an ulnar styloid fracture.

- Transradial variants include a radial styloid fracture.

- Transcapitate variants include a capitate neck fracture. The detached capitate head usually rotates, often a full 180°.

- Whenever scaphoid waist fractures are widely displaced, an associated midcarpal joint disruption or other ligament injury should be suspected.

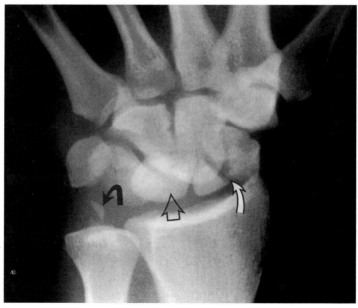

A

FIGURE 21   Trans-scapho-perilunate dislocation. This is the most common of all intercarpal dislocations. **(A)** The PA view shows the displaced scaphoid fracture *(curved white arrow)*, an ulnar styloid fracture *(curved black arrow)*, an abnormally shaped lunate *(open arrow)*, and overlap of the proximal and distal carpal rows.

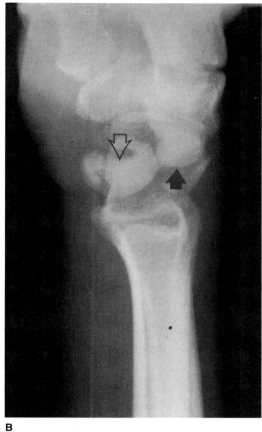

FIGURE 21

(B) The lateral view shows that the lunate *(open arrow)* is no longer articulating with the head of the capitate *(closed arrow).*

B

Suggested Reading

Yin Y, Mann FA, Gilula LA. In: Gilula LA, Yin Y. eds. *Imaging of the Wrist and Hand.* Philadelphia: WB Saunders; 1996:93–157.

Rogers LF. In: *Radiology of Skeletal Trauma.* New York: Churchill Livingstone; 1992: 911–929.

Radiographically Occult Fractures Detected by Bone Scan

KEY FACTS

- Occult fractures are detected because of the osteoblastic response shown by bone scan. Eighty percent will be positive on scan within 24 hours of the event.

- Planar imaging is sensitive, but SPECT is more so, particularly in the spine due to enhanced lesion contrast.

- In older individuals, >75 years, if the initial scan is negative, a repeat scan in 48 to 72 hours is usually revealing of the injury.

- The bone scan is a way of screening the entire skeletal system for the effects of trauma or other occult disease.

- Bone scan is a method for evaluating victims of abuse.

- In sports medicine, the bone scan detects stress fractures and other sports-related injuries to bone.

- Stress fractures may be detected by bone scan much earlier than radiography, which sometimes requires approximately 1 to 3 weeks after injury, a period during which periosteal reaction may appear.

- Stress fractures can be graded from I to IV on the size and characteristics of radionuclide uptake in bone, from periosteal reaction only, to true fracture that extends 50% or more into the cortex. Lesser grades take a shorter time to heal.

- Other entities may make bone scanning non-specific for fractures such as: co-existent osteomyelitis, metastatic disease, and also heterotopic ossification, although the latter categories have scan patterns that may render more specific diagnoses by experienced interpreters.

- The earliest time in which a bone scan will return to normal after a fracture is about 5 months.

- Ninety percent of fractures will have a normal appearance on bone scan by 2 years after the event.

- Another latent effect of injury is well documented by the triple phase bone scan: reflex sympathetic dystrophy.

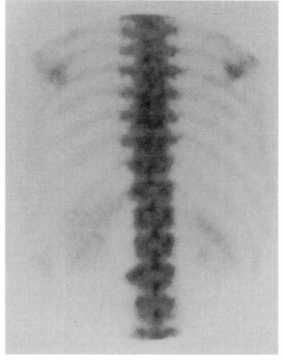

A

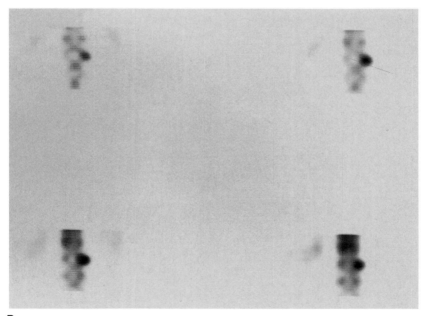

B

F I G U R E   2 2   **(A)** Planar bone image with Tc-99m medronate of lumbar spine showing abnormality at L-3. **(B)** SPECT image enhances contrast of the lesion so that it is more readily detectable. This was a transverse process fracture in a man with continued back pain after an industrial accident.

Part C: Upper Extremity

Radiographically Occult Fractures Detected by Bone Scan *(Continued)*

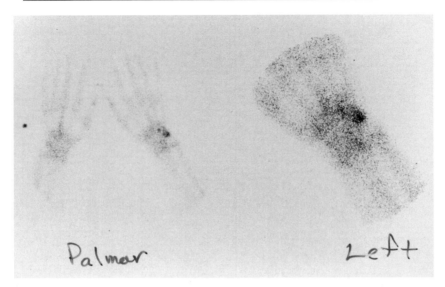

FIGURE 23   Planar wrist image showing left triquetral and hamate fracture in a soccer player who performed a bicycle kick and complained of left wrist pain.

Suggested Reading
Collier BD Jr, Fogelman I, Brown ML. Bone scintigraphy: Part 2. Orthopedic bone scanning. *J Nucl Med.* 1993;34(12):2241–2246.

Metacarpal Fractures

KEY FACTS

- Metacarpal fractures are classified by their location: Base, shaft, neck, or head.

- Metacarpal base fractures involve the carpometatcarpal joints. They are most common at the thumb metacarpal base.

- First metacarpal base fractures are classified according to the pattern of articular involvement. They are known as Bennett's (Figure 24), Rolando's (Figure 25), and extra-articular (Figure 26) fractures.

- Bennett's fracture (Figure 24) has a small palmar detached fragment, usually with proximal displacement of the remainder of the metacarpal.

- Rolando's fracture (Figure 25) has both palmar and dorsal detached fragments.

- Metacarpal shaft fractures are usually the result of more indirect trauma and are either transverse or oblique (Figure 28). The direction of the fracture depending on the direction of the force—either bending or twisting.

- Metacarpal neck fractures are the result of direct blows to the metacarpal head, usually with the fist clenched. These fractures are usually unstable, with palmar angulation and/or displacement of the metacarpal head.

- The fifth metacarpal neck is fractured most commonly (Figure 27), followed by the second metacarpal neck. These fractures both result from punching.

- Rotational deformity can occur with both shaft and neck fractures. This results in significant morbidity as it interferes with the ability of the hand to grip or make a fist.

- Metacarpal head fractures are intra-articular and can lead to long-term joint sequelae, such as osteoarthritis.

Metacarpal Fractures (Continued)

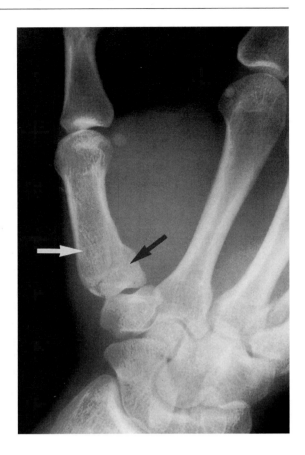

FIGURE 24

Bennett's fracture. This articular fracture of the first metatarsal base has a large palmar retained fragment *(black arrow)* with minimal proximal displacement of the remainder of the bone *(white arrow)*.

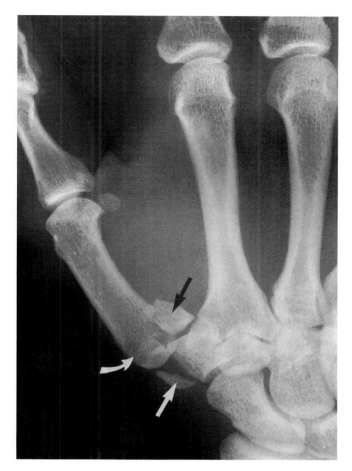

FIGURE 25   Rolando's fracture. This articular fracture of the first metatarsal base has both palmar *(black arrow)* and dorsal *(white arrow)* fragments with minimal proximal displacement of the remainder of the bone *(curved white arrow).*

Metacarpal Fractures (Continued)

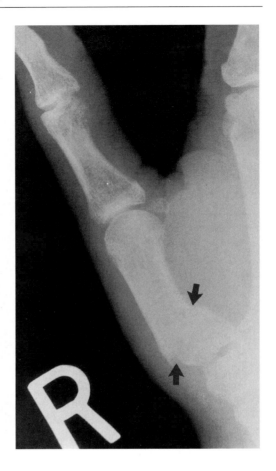

FIGURE 26

Extra-articular first metacarpal base fracture. This angulated fracture *(arrows)* is situated well distal to the articular surface. The distal portion of the bone is displaced proximally.

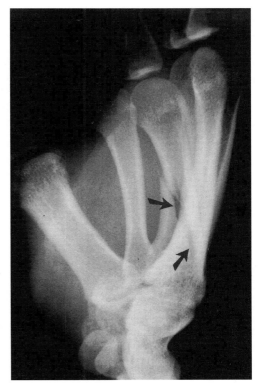

A

FIGURE 27

Fourth metacarpal shaft fracture. This fracture is usually caused by a blow to the closed fist. In this patient the fracture *(arrows)* was only visible on **(A)** the lateral view. It was not seen on **(B)** the PA view or **(C)** the oblique view. Another illustration of the need for multiple views in extremity fractures. The most serious deformity in these spiral fractures is rotation, which is more reliably assessed clinically than radiologically.

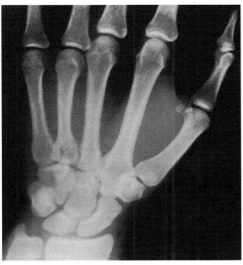

B

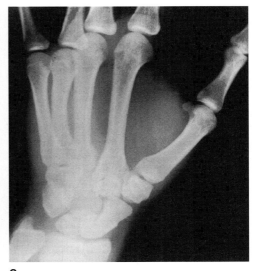

C

Metacarpal Fractures (Continued)

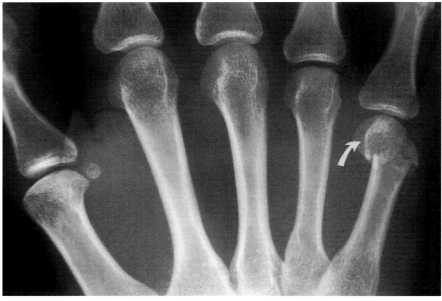

A

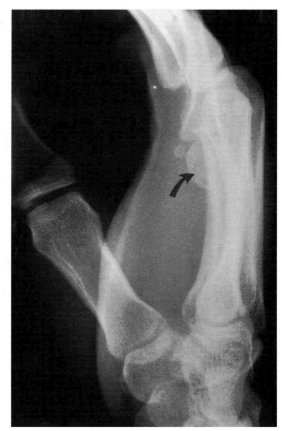

B

FIGURE 28

Boxer's fracture. This patient punched a wall and sustained a slightly comminuted fracture of the fifth metacarpal neck. **(A)** PA and **(B)** lateral views show that the distal fracture fragment *(arrows)* is angulated palmarly and is slightly rotated. As with spiral shaft fractures, the rotation is the most significant deformity.

Suggested Reading

Green DP, Towland SA. In: Rockwood CA, Green DP, Bucholz RW. eds. *Rockwood and Green's Fractures*. Philadelphia: Lippincott; 1991:441–500.

Trumble TE, Stack JT. In: Hansen ST, Swiontkowski MF. eds. *Orthopaedic Trauma Protocols*. New York: Raven Press; 1993:153–185.

Phalangeal Fractures

KEY FACTS

- The commonest finger bone to be fractured is the distal phalanx. These bones are typically crushed, resulting in a comminuted but minimally displaced fracture of the terminal tuft.

- Open injuries to the distal phalanx are not infrequent. In these injuries, portions of the phalanx are often lost.

- Avulsion of the extensor tendon from the base of the distal phalanx occurs as a result of a blow to the end of an extended finger. The characteristic deformity is persistent flexion of the distal interphalangeal joint—known as a mallet deformity.

- Mallet deformities are often associated with avulsion fractures of the dorsal lip of the base of the distal phalanx.

- Hyperextension injuries can avulse the cartilaginous volar plate (into which the short flexor tendon inserts) from the palmar aspect of the base of the middle phalanx. This usually results in a small fragment of bone being avulsed from the phalanx (Figure 29).

- True lateral views of the injured fingers (without overlapping fingers) are essential to show the small avulsion fractures associated with mallet and volar plate injuries.

- Abduction injuries to the thumb result in avulsion of the ulnar collateral ligament from the base of the proximal phalanx. This injury, known as "gamekeeper's thumb," usually includes a small fragment of bone and may involve the articular surface (Figure 30).

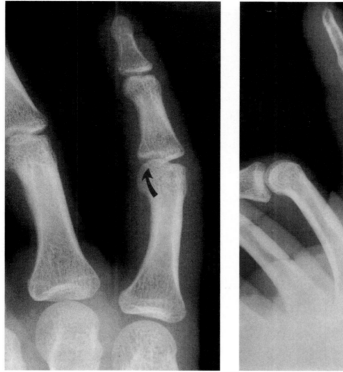

A

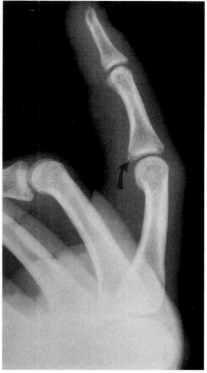

B

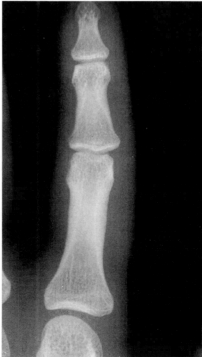

C

FIGURE 29

Volar plate fracture. **(A)** Oblique and **(B)** lateral views of the little finger show a small avulsed fragment *(arrows)* at the base of the proximal phalanx. As with most of these injuries, the fracture cannot be seen on **(C)** the PA view. The lateral view is essential to show displacement, and often is the only view on which the fracture can be identified.

Part C: Upper Extremity

Phalangeal Fractures (Continued)

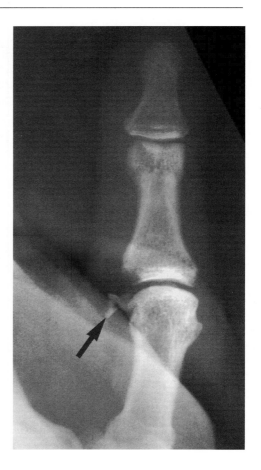

FIGURE 30

Gamekeeper's thumb. AP view of the thumb showing a small piece of bone *(arrow)* that has been avulsed from the ulnar aspect of the base of the proximal phalanx. This fragment is markedly displaced. It represents an avulsion of the ulnar collateral ligament and the metacarpophalangeal joint is almost certainly unstable when the fragment is displaced this much.

Suggested Reading

Green DP, Towland SA. In: Rockwood CA, Green DP, Bucholz RW. eds. *Rockwood and Green's Fractures*. Philadelphia: Lippincott; 1991:500–542.

Trumble TE, Sack JT. In: Hansen ST, Swiontkowski MF. eds. *Orthopaedic Trauma Protocols*. New York: Raven Press; 1993:153–185.

PELVIS/LOWER EXTREMITY

Pelvic Apophyseal Avulsions

KEY FACTS

- Pelvic apophyseal injuries are the result of a forceful muscular pull, usually secondary to athletic activities.

- These injuries usually occur in adolescents before closure of the apophysis; the muscle and tendon are stronger than their apophyseal attachment.

- These avulsions are often initially diagnosed as a "muscle pull."

- When acute, the origin of the fracture fragment is usually obvious on radiographs. However, if initial imaging is delayed into the healing phase, more ominous diagnoses, such as tumor, may be considered leading to unnecessary and at times disastrous biopsies if the healing fracture is misinterpreted as a sarcoma.

- The pelvic apophyses and their associated muscles are:
    - Iliac crest: abdominal muscles (avulsion known as "hip pointer")
    - Anterior superior iliac spine: sartorius
    - Anterior inferior iliac spine: rectus femoris
    - Ischial tuberosity: biceps femoris (hamstrings)

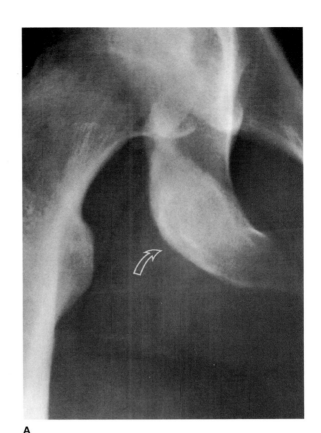

A

FIGURE 1

Ischial avulsion fracture: A 38-year-old martial arts aficionado complained of pain in the hip region following a vigorous workout involving kicking. AP radiograph **(A)** shows a very subtle bony fragment *(curved arrow)* adjacent to the right ischial tuberosity. Axial CT scan through the same area **(B)** shows the avulsed fragment of ischium *(arrow),* presumably secondary to hamstring muscle avulsion.

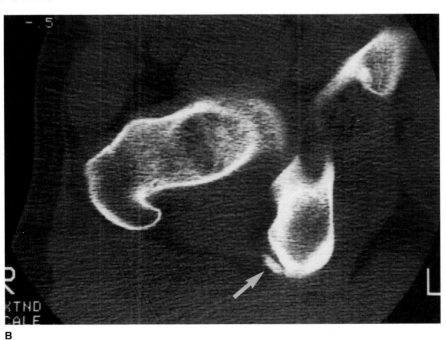

B

Suggested Reading

Rogers LF. *Radiology of Skeletal Trauma*. 2nd ed. New York: Churchill Livingstone; 1992:1080–1086.

Lateral Compression Pelvic Fracture

KEY FACTS

- Lateral compression refers to an internal rotation injury resulting from a blow to the side of the pelvis, such as when an automobile is broadsided.

- The lateral compression fracture is the most common pattern encountered in most series, accounting for 60% to 70% of pelvic ring fractures.

- Horizontal or coronal plane obturator ring fractures are noted in nearly every case. They tend to overlap.

- A "buckle" type fracture of the sacral ala, often extending inferiorly into the sacrum is seen in nearly 90% of cases.

- The sacral fracture may be quite subtle on conventional radiographs, with only minimal asymmetry of the involved ala or disruption of arcuate lines of the sacrum. However, the sacral fracture is obvious on CT scan.

- Internal rotation of the pelvis may be evident on conventional radiograph or CT examination.

- The pubic symphysis and SI joints are spared.

- Complex or combined mechanisms are common. One pattern of interest is the so-called "windswept pelvis," an external rotation (anterior compression) injury on one side and an internal rotation (lateral compression) injury on the contralateral side.

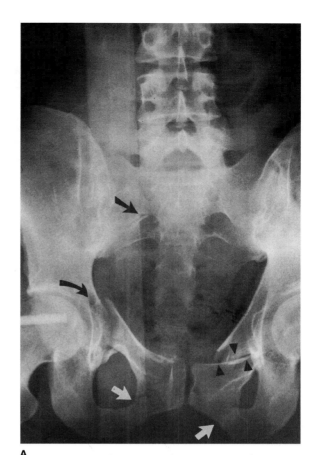

FIGURE 2

Lateral compression fractures: Two patients. **(A)** Patient 1. AP pelvis shows horizontally oriented overlapping fractures of the left superior and inferior pubic rami on the left *(black arrowheads, superior; white arrow, inferior)*. Fractures of the right root of the superior ramus *(curved black arrow)* and inferior ramus at the pubis *(white arrow)* were also seen. The arcuate line of the right S1 foramen *(diagonal black arrow)* is not continuous (compare to left) indicating sacral fracture. **(B)** Patient 2. The buckling fracture of the upper sacrum may subtle on plain radiographs, but CT will show the lesion as on this axial image *(arrow)*.

A

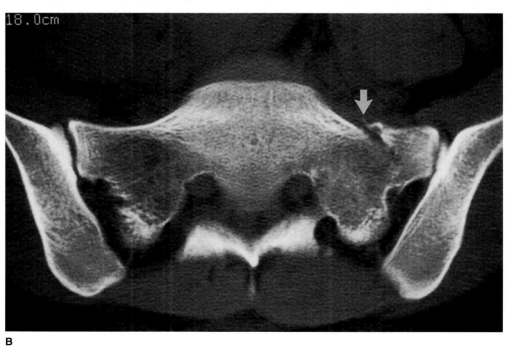

B

Suggested Reading

Daffner RH. Pelvic trauma. In: McCort JJ, Mindelzun RE. ed. *Trauma Radiology*. New York: Churchill Livingstone; 1990:339–380.

Anterior Compression Pelvic Fracture

KEY FACTS

- Anterior compression pelvic fracture is the result of a force applied either directly to the anterior or to the posterior pelvis and results in varying degrees of "open book" or iliac external rotation deformity.

- Anterior compression pelvic fracture accounts for 15% of pelvic ring fractures and is intermediate in frequency between lateral compression and vertical shear injuries.

- Diastasis of both the symphysis pubis and sacroiliac (SI) joint are the hallmark of this fracture pattern.

- The greater the separation of the symphysis pubis, the greater the implied ligamentous damage and hence, the unstable nature of the fracture.

- Obturator ring fractures are variable and usually indicative of a direct blow to the symphysis.

- CT scanning of the SI joints can show disruption anteriorly with intact posterior articulation in the more stable types.

- Widening of the posterior sacroiliac joints implies disruption of the important posterior sacroiliac ligaments and a more unstable injury.

- Determination of pelvic stability, in our institution, is primarily a clinical decision, with the imaging used as an adjunct.

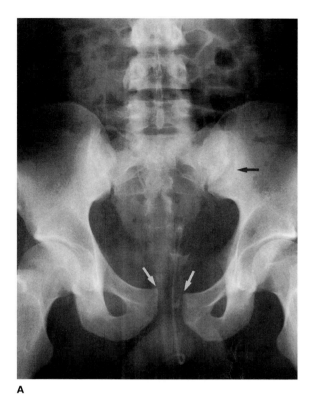

FIGURE 3

Anterior compression fractures: Two patients. **(A)** Widening of the symphysis pubis *(white arrows)* and left sacroiliac (SI) joint *(black arrow)* are the hallmark of this fracture pattern. A urethral catheter is in the bladder with some residual contrast from cystography. **(B)** Another patient with symphyseal diastasis *(white arrows)* and minimal widening of both SI joints *(black arrows)*.(See Both Column Acetabular Fracture, Figure 10C.)

A

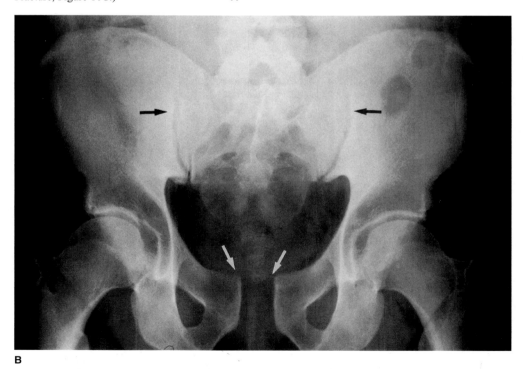

B

Suggested Reading

Kellam JF, Browner BD. Fractures of the pelvic ring. In: Browner BD, Jupiter JB, Levine AM, Trafton PG. ed. *Skeletal Trauma*. Philadelphia: WB Saunders; 1992:849–897.

Vertical Shear Pelvic Fracture

KEY FACTS

- The mechanism of injury involves an asymmetric axial load on the pelvis, often transmitted through the ipsilateral lower extremity.
- Vertical shear pelvic fractures account for 6% to 13% of pelvic ring fractures.
- The characteristic finding in all cases of vertical shear pelvic fracture is superior displacement of the involved hemipelvis with respect to the opposite side on conventional radiographs.
- The outlet view is useful to confirm superior displacement of the involved hemipelvis.
- Anteriorly, fractures of the pubic rami are usually noted.
- Posterior disruption of the pelvis usually involves sacral fracture, with sacroiliac diastasis or iliac wing fracture as notable variants.
- At times, disruption of the symphysis pubis and sacroiliac joint are noted without fracture and displacement of the pelvis occurs through these structures.

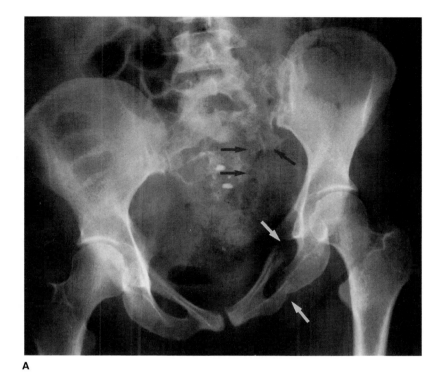

A

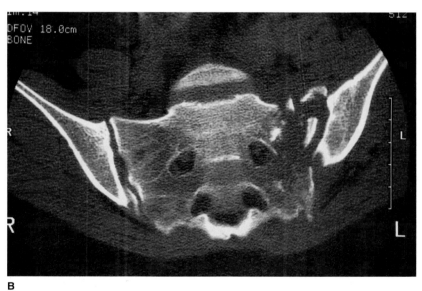

B

FIGURE 4 Vertical shear fracture: **(A)** AP pelvis radiograph shows upward displacement of the left hemipelvis compared to the right (note position of left hip and top of iliac crest). Fractures through the left obturator ring *(white arrows)* and left sacrum *(black arrows)* allow this displacement in this typical vertical shear fracture. **(B)** Direct coronal CT scan shows the fractures of the left sacrum extending into the left SI joint, but spare the sacral foramina (zone I fracture). (See discussion of Sacral Fracture for discussion of the Denis classification.)

Suggested Reading

Young JWR, Burgess AR, Brumbach RJ, Poka A. Pelvic fractures: Value of plain radiography in early assessment and management. *Radiology.* 1986;160:445–451.

Pelvic Ring Disruption and Arterial Injury

KEY FACTS

- The most common mechanisms for pelvic ring disruptions are motor vehicle accidents (48%), auto versus pedestrian (18%), falls (14%), motorcycle accidents (11%), crush injuries (4%), and miscellaneous (5%). Mortality varies from 5% to 50%, and correlates with the Injury Severity Score and the age of the patient. The majority of associated deaths are due to hemorrhage.

- Many classification schemes have been developed to predict the likelihood of mortality and hemorrhage related to pelvic ring disruptions. Most commonly used is the modified Young and Burgess classification, which is based on the major vector force of injury: anterior-posterior (AP) compression (Types I, II, II), lateral compression (Types I, II, III), vertical shear and combined mechanical.

- Sources of pelvic hemorrhage include arteries, veins and osseous structures.

- Modalities for treating pelvic hemorrhage include pneumatic anti-shock garment, external fixation, surgical exploration and ligation and angiographic embolization. External fixation controls hemorrhage from osseous, venous, and minor arterial origins.

- Arterial bleeding is usually from internal iliac artery branches; frequency in descending order are superior gluteal, internal pudendal, lateral sacral, and obturator arteries.

- There is a high frequency of arterial hemorrhage in AP compression (Types II, III), vertical shear, combined mechanical, crushed fracture of the sacrum, and any fracture extending to the greater sciatic notch. Neither conservative management by blood volume replacement nor aggressive management by surgical exploration and ligation of the internal iliac arteries has proven successful in controlling arterial hemorrhage. Bilateral internal iliac artery ligation usually fail because the extensive pelvic collaterals prevent the isolation of the bleeding site. Furthermore, decompression of the hematoma may release its tamponade effect leading to intraoperative death from exsanguination.

- Transcatheter embolization is utilized to control arterial hemorrhage. Seven to eleven percent of the patients undergoing angiography may require embolization; 1.7% in simple lateral compression and 20% in AP compression, vertical shear and combined mechanical. Transcatheter embolization, with gelfoam and/or coils, should be performed in all cases of arterial injury manifesting as contrast extravasation, abrupt or tapered occlusion and pseudoaneurysm. A temporary occlusion balloon can be placed for active bleeding from transected common iliac, external iliac or common femoral artery. The patient can then be transported for emergency surgical repair.

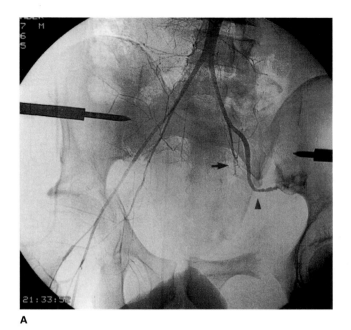

A

B

FIGURE 5   29-year-old man run over by a backhoe had a large left groin hematoma and underwent external fixation of his pelvic ring disruption. The patient remained hemodynamically unstable, with falling serial hematocrit values. Note widening of the left sacroiliac joint, displaced left obturator ring fracture, diastasis of the pubic symphysis and a right acetabular fracture **(A)**. Early **(A)** And late **(B)** arterial phase of nonselective pelvic arteriogram performed via right common femoral artery access shows multiple occlusions of the proximal branches of the left internal iliac artery *(arrow)*, probably secondary to transection, and complete disruption of the left external iliac artery with frank extravasation of contrast *(arrowhead)*. An occlusion balloon was introduced and inflated in the distal aorta, at its bifurcation, to decrease bleeding prior to surgical repair.

Suggested Reading

Ben-Menachem Y, Coldwell DM, Young JWR, Burgess AR. Hemorrhage associated with pelvic ring disruptions: Causes, diagnosis, and emergent management. *AJR*. 1991;157: 1005–1014.

Sacral Fracture

KEY FACTS

- Fewer than 5% of sacral fractures occur as isolated injuries. Most are associated with pelvic or lumbar spine fractures.

- Sacral fractures are usually vertical in orientation, with only 5% to 10% occurring in the transverse plane.

- High transverse fractures are seen at the S1 or S2 level are usually secondary to a high energy injury such as a fall. They tend to show kyphosis and overriding on the lateral radiograph.

- Low transverse fractures (S3 or S4) are usually due to a direct blow with a fracture at the level of the lower end of the SI joints. Both types of transverse sacral fracture are frequently associated with neurologic deficit.

- Using plain radiographs and CT, approximately 90% of pelvic fractures are have associated sacral injury.

- One useful classification is the Denis Classification which divides the sacrum into three zones:
  - Zone I. Lateral to foramina: 50% of cases, 6% neurologic deficits
  - Zone II. Transforaminal: 34% of cases, 28% neurologic deficits
  - Zone III. Central canal involvement: 8% of cases, 57% neurologic deficits

- Plain radiographs detect only 30% of sacral fractures; another 35% can be seen in retrospect. Transverse sacral fractures are difficult to see on frontal plain films and careful analysis of the lateral is essential. On the AP radiographs, fracture lines and displacements are sought. Disruption of the **arcuate lines**, the dense cortical arcs outlining the roof of each sacral foramen is a useful sign of sacral fracture.

- We perform CT for any recognized or suspected sacral fracture or sacroiliac disruption. CT is superior to plain radiographs in detecting sacral fractures. Care must be exercised with transverse injuries, whose fracture lines may parallel the scanning plane and missed without multiplanar reformations.

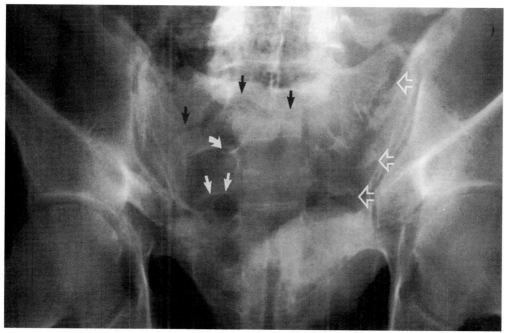

A

B

FIGURE 6

(A) Outlet view of the pelvis (AP with 45° of cephalad angulation) shows a transverse fracture of the sacrum through the S1 foramina *(black arrows)* disruption of the right S2 arcuate line *(curved white arrow)* and a vertical fracture through the left sacrum *(open white arrows)*. Compare the normal arcuate line of S3 on the right *(white arrows)*. (B) Lateral lumbosacral spine radiograph shows the fracture through the S1-S2 level, kyphosis and overriding *(arrows)*. *(continued)*

Sacral Fracture (Continued)

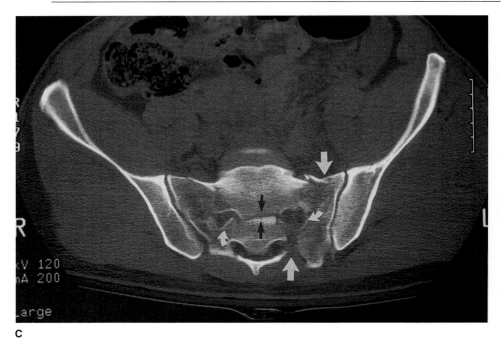

C

F I G U R E 6 (CONTINUED)   **(C)** Axial CT scan through the sacrum shows the vertical *(white arrows)* and horizontal *(black arrows)* components of this H-shaped fracture. Asymmetry of the foramina *(curved arrows)* is highlighted.

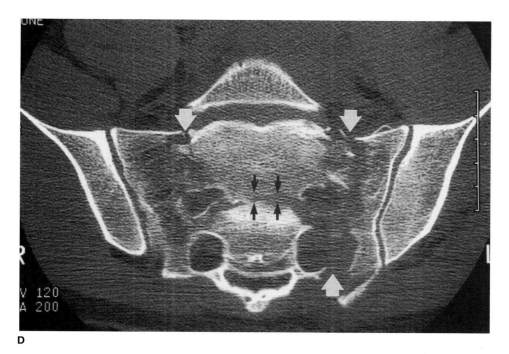

D

F I G U R E 6 **(D)** direct coronal CT scan through the sacrum shows the vertical *(white arrows)* and horizontal *(black arrows)* components of this H-shaped fracture. Asymmetry of the foramina *(curved arrows)* is highlighted.

Suggested Reading

Levine AM. Lumbar and sacral spine trauma. In: Browner BD, Jupiter JB, Levine AM, Trafton PG, ed. *Skeletal Trauma*. Philadelphia: WB Saunders;1992:1959–1991.

Anterior Hip Dislocation

KEY FACTS

- These injuries account for approximately 10% of hip dislocations.
- The mechanism of injury involves forced abduction and external rotation.
- Anterior dislocations are usually displaced inferomedial, often projecting over the obturator ring on the AP pelvic radiograph.
- Femoral head injuries are common, with an acetabular rim fracture occurring less commonly than with posterior hip dislocations. CT scans often show injuries to the femoral head and rim better than conventional radiographs.
- CT scanning is indicated for all hip dislocations. CT is the optimal procedure to evaluate the joint space including joint congruity, retained osseous fragments, and associated acetabular or femoral head fractures.
- Failure to obtain an anatomic reduction of the joint should suggest entrapped fragments or interposed cartilaginous labrum. If the CT scan does not show ossified loose fragments, CT arthrotomography with air may be useful for detecting cartilaginous bodies or a displaced labrum.

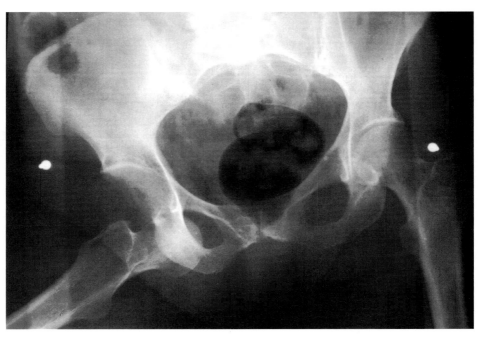

FIGURE 7   AP pelvis view demonstrates an anterior dislocation of the right hip. The femoral head overlies the right obturator ring.

Suggested Reading

Levin P. Hip dislocations. In: Browner BD, Jupiter JB, Levine AM, Trafton PG. eds. *Skeletal Trauma*. Philadelphia: WB Saunders; 1992:1329–1367.

Basic Acetabular Anatomy

KEY FACTS

- The pelvis has been likened to the an inverted "Y," with the vertical limb being the ilium, the lower, anterior, and posterior limbs being the respective columns, and the acetabulum lying at their intersection.

- The *anterior column* consists of the anterior aspect of the ilium wing, pelvic brim, superior pubic ramus, anterior wall of the acetabulum, and the teardrop.

- The *posterior column* consists of the posterior ilium, the posterior articular surface and posterior wall of the acetabulum, the ischium and most of the quadrilateral plate (medial acetabular wall).

- Acetabular imaging begins with AP and Judet views of the pelvis; the latter films are 45° anterior and posterior oblique views of the involved hemipelvis. CT is indicated in all complex acetabular fractures to complete the workup.

- Basic observations on the radiographs include detection of the fractures and localization the appropriate column or wall.

- On the AP radiograph, column markers are:
  - Anterior column-*iliopectineal line,* the pelvic brim
  - Posterior column-*ilioischial line,* formed by the posterior quadrilateral plate

- On the Judet views:
  - The posterior (iliac) oblique shows the anterior wall and posterior column to best advantage
  - The anterior (obturator) oblique shows the posterior wall and anterior column to best advantage

- Basic observations on CT scans include localization of the fracture to the appropriate wall or column, evaluation of the articular weight-bearing surface, detection of intra-articular entrapped fragments, and femoral head injury.

Suggested Reading

Letournel E, Judet R. *Fractures of the Acetabulum.* 2nd ed. New York: Springer-Verlag; 1993.

Posterior Hip Dislocation

KEY FACTS

- Posterior dislocations account for approximately 90% of hip dislocations; the other 10% are anterior. A central dislocation refers to displacement of the femoral head into the pelvis via a break in the medial wall of the acetabulum. This term is not favored by orthopaedic surgeons because the injury really represents an acetabular fracture.

- The mechanism of injury in 70% to 100% of cases involves the knee striking the dashboard during a motor-vehicle accident, frequently involving unrestrained occupants, thus forcing the femoral head posteriorly.

- Femoral head injuries occur as the femoral head exits the acetabulum. Avulsions from the ligamentum teres also occur.

- Complications of a posterior hip dislocation include:
  - Osteoarthritis secondary to articular cartilage injury or retained loose fragments
  - Osteonecrosis:
    - Reported incidence varies from 1% to 15% with an average of 10%
    - Delay in reduction is considered an important etiologic factor

- Associated injuries include those typical of high energy trauma: central nervous system, cardiovascular, lung and chest wall, visceral and other musculoskeletal injuries. Ipsilateral lower extremity, hip, and acetabular fractures must be excluded.

- Radiographic hallmarks include:
  - Superior and lateral displacement of the femoral head
  - Involved femoral head smaller (closer to film) than the contralateral hip on AP pelvis radiograph
  - Internal rotation of femur

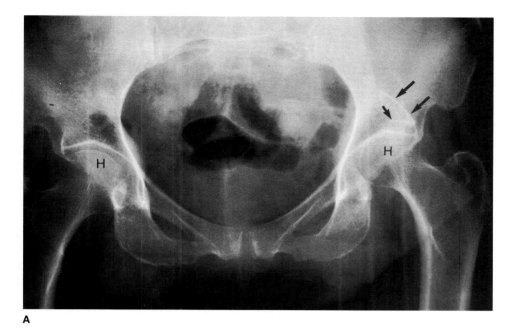

A

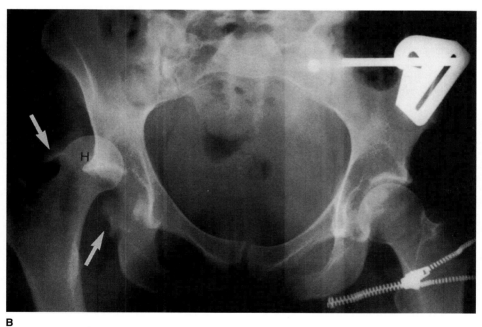

B

F I G U R E 8   Three patients. **(A)** Patient 1 with left posterior hip dislocation. Compare the sizes of the femoral heads (H)—the left appears smaller since it is closer to the film. A triangular piece of posterior acetabular wall *(arrows)* is seen above the head *(arrows)*. Patient 2: AP radiograph of the pelvis **(B)**. *(continued)*

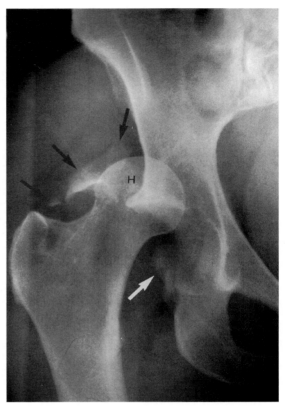

FIGURE 8 (CONTINUED)
(C) Patient 2: Close-up of the right hip shows superior displacement of the right femoral head (H), superiorly displaced posterior wall fragments *(arrows)* and comminuted fracture of the remainder of the posterior wall *(arrows)*. **(D)** Patient 3 had a left posterior hip dislocation that would not reduce concentrically . Axial CT through the left hip shows lateral displacement of the femoral head (H) by an entrapped fragment of posterior wall *(white arrow)* in the anterior half of the joint space. The large defect in the posterior wall *(black arrows)* is seen as well. GT = the top of the greater trochanter.

C

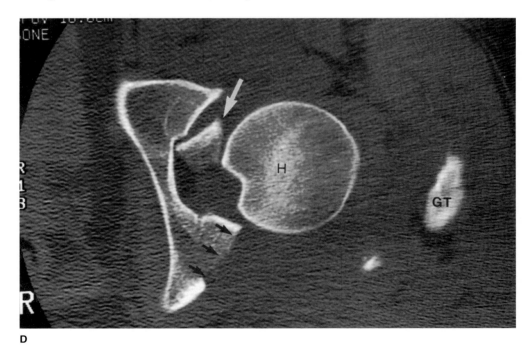

D

Suggested Reading

Levin P. Hip dislocations. In: Browner BD, Jupiter JB, Levine AM, Trafton PG. ed. *Skeletal Trauma*. Philadelphia: WB Saunders; 1992:1329–1367.

Posterior Wall Acetabular Fracture

KEY FACTS

- About one third of acetabular fractures involve the posterior wall, and are usually associated with posterior dislocation of the hip.

- Associated femoral head injury, usually either an impaction fracture or a shearing injury, is noted in 12% of posterior dislocations. It may be subtle and best seen on CT.

- Focal compression of the acetabular articular surface, or marginal impaction, ("die-punch" fracture) is seen in about one quarter of posterior dislocations and is seen best on axial CT scans. Preoperative diagnosis of marginal impaction is essential for surgical planning; treatment includes elevation of the depression and placement of bone graft in any residual defect.

- Forty-five percent of patients with posterior wall fractures have associated fractures elsewhere in the skeleton, often in the femoral neck or shaft and adjacent pelvis.

- Associated injuries include:
  - Sciatic nerve injury in 12% of patients
  - Laceration of the superior gluteal artery
  - Avascular necrosis of the femoral head in 8% to 10% of patients, usually occurring 3 to 18 months following dislocation

Suggested Reading

Matta J. Surgical treatment of acetabular fractures. In: Browner BD, Jupiter JB, Levine AM, Trafton PG. ed. *Skeletal Trauma*. Philadelphia: WB Saunders; 1992:899–922.

Transverse Acetabular Fracture

KEY FACTS

- The term "transverse" can be confusing, but is based on the original anatomic description of Judet and Letournel, viewing the acetabulum from a lateral perspective. On CT scanning, the fracture is oriented from anterior to posterior in the sagittal plane.

- While this fracture involves the anterior and posterior columns, it is not a both column fracture—this is a different injury.

- Transverse fractures:
  - Sagittal plane on CT scan through the tectum (roof)
  - Acetabular roof remains attached to the ilium and ipsilateral sacroiliac joint

- Both column fractures:
  - Coronal plane on CT scan through the tectum (roof)
  - Loss of continuity between the acetabular roof and ilium/SI joint

- Transverse fractures are elementary or simple lesions in the Letournel-Judet classification. However, complex variations occur such as the T-type and transverse-posterior wall patterns. Overall, transverse fractures and its variants account for approximately one third of acetabular fractures.

- A T-Type fracture is a transverse fracture with a vertical component. An inferior ramus fracture in association with a transverse pattern on conventional radiographs or the presence of a fracture of the medial wall of the acetabulum (quadrilateral plate) on CT scan is noted in this fracture pattern.

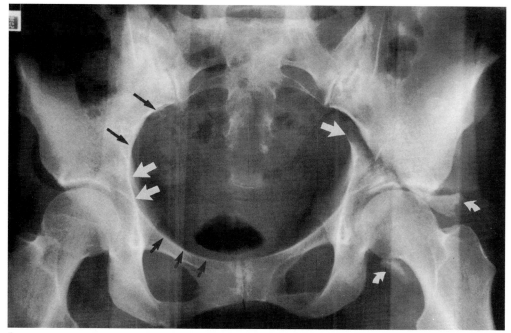

A

B

FIGURE 9

AP pelvis **(A)** and obturator (anterior) oblique Judet **(B)** radiographs show a fracture of the left acetabulum disrupting the ilioischial line in **(A)** *(left white arrow),* and the iliopectineal line in **(A)** and **(B)** (*black arrow* in B). On the normal right side, white arrows show the ilioischial line, black arrows the iliopectineal line. A comminuted fracture of the posterior wall of the acetabulum is present with fragments above and below the acetabulum (*arrows,* A and B). *(continued)*

Transverse Acetabular Fracture *(Continued)*

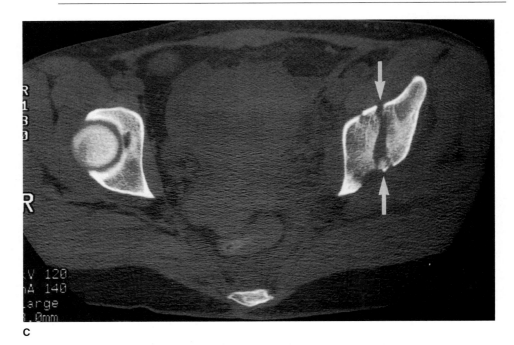

C

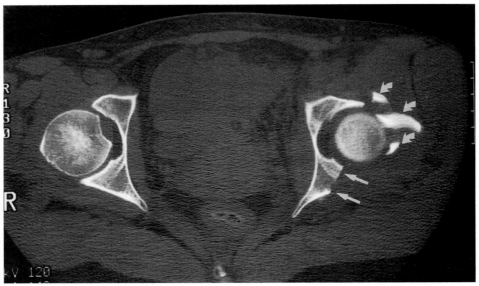

D

F I G U R E   9 (CONTINUED)   **(C)** Axial CT scan through the tectum (roof) of the left acetabulum show the typical anterior-posterior orientation of the transverse fracture pattern *(white arrows)*. **(D)** Axial CT scan through the hip joints show the obliquely oriented posterior wall fracture *(white arrows)* and multiple displaced fragments of the posterior wall *(curved arrows)*.

Suggested Reading
Brandser EA, El-Khoury GY, Marsh JL. Acetabular fractures: A systematic approach to classification. *Emergency Radiology*. 1995;2(1):18–28.

Both Column Acetabular Fracture

KEY FACTS

- The both column acetabular fracture is the most common of the complex acetabular fracture patterns and accounts for 20% to 25% of all acetabular fractures.

- In this fracture the acetabulum is dissociated from the intact ilium and its sacroiliac attachments. The acetabulum is essentially floating free, usually displaced medially into the pelvis. It is highly unstable and usually requires surgical reduction.

- This pattern needs to be distinguished from the transverse fracture pattern, since the surgical approach is different for each type. Both fractures involve the anterior and posterior columns of the acetabulum, but the fracture patterns are distinct (see Transverse Acetabular Fracture discussion).

- The hallmark of the both column fracture is the "spur sign" on the obturator oblique Judet view (injured side rotated up 45°).

- The spur represents the part of the ilium that remains attached to the sacrum at the SI joint. Following the ilium caudally on CT scanning, it does not attach to the tectum, or roof, of the acetabulum, confirming the diagnosis.

- In general, column fractures (i.e., anterior, posterior, both column) are in the coronal plane on CT scans through the roof of the acetabulum. Contrast the orientation of the posterior acetabular wall and transverse acetabular fractures in following sections. CT scans through the tectum of the acetabulum in fractures of the anterior or posterior wall are oblique in orientation, while transverse fractures are oriented in an anteroposterior direction.

Both Column Acetabular Fracture (Continued)

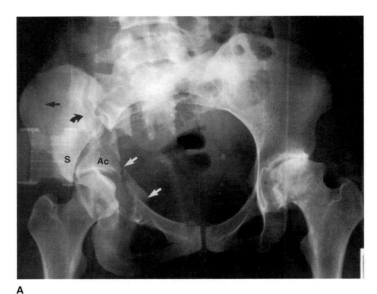

A

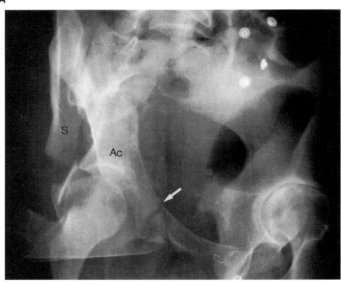

B

F I G U R E   1 0   (A) AP pelvis film shows a right acetabular fracture in a 26-year-old patient with undocumented childhood left hip problem and resultant degenerative change. Separation of the anterior and posterior columns of the acetabulum has allowed the right hip joint to displace medially into the pelvis. The line of separation *(arrows)* of the acetabulum (Ac) from the ilium and its attachments to the sacroiliac joint ends distally in a sharp spur of bone (S) and accounts for the spur sign on the obturator oblique view **(B).** Other findings in **(A)** include an iliac wing fracture *(black arrow)* and widening of the right SI joint *(curved arrow).* **(B)** The obturator oblique view (45° left posterior oblique) shows the spur sign (S); the spur represents the stable part of the ilium that remains attached to the SI joint with the acetabulum (Ac) floating free. The anterior column fracture is indicated by the disruption of the iliopectineal line (*white arrows* in A and B). **(C)–(E)** Axial CT scans of the pelvis with (S) representing the spur seen on **(B).** On successive scans note that the spur is not continuous with the tectum (or roof) (T) in **(E)** of the acetabulum, the hallmark of the both column fracture. The fracture line through the acetabulum is horizontal or coronal in orientation, typical of column fractures *(arrow).* Widening of the anterior right sacroiliac joint is seen in **(C).**

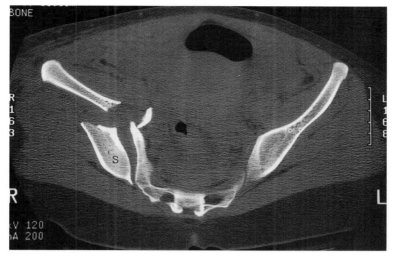

C

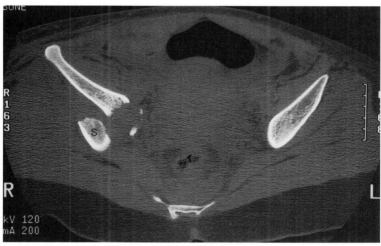

D

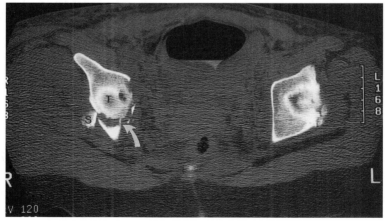

E

Suggested Reading

Letournel E, Judet R. *Fractures of the Acetabulum*. 2nd ed. New York: Springer-Verlag; 1993.

Acetabular Fracture: Indications for Angiography

KEY FACTS

- Acetabular fractures usually result from high energy trauma, such as motor-vehicle accidents and falls. In the classification of Judet and Letournel used by most pelvic surgeons, simple (elementary) fractures occur in 40% of patients, while complex (associated) injuries are seen in the remainder. The accurate classification of these injuries is essential for treatment planning.

- Anteroposterior views of the pelvis and Judet oblique views are the initial means of assessing these fractures. These conventional radiographs can define the fracture type in most cases; however, the orientation, location and exact number of fracture fragments, as well as, the status of the joint space requires CT scanning. Two- and three-dimensional reformations are often used for surgical planning in complex injuries.

- Pre-operative angiography of a complex acetabular fracture can be helpful if the fracture involves the greater sciatic notch, when fracture fragment(s) are displaced into the greater sciatic notch, or if the patient has unexplained hypotension. Acetabular fractures that involve the greater sciatic notch have a high incidence of superior gluteal artery injury. It is important to localize and embolize injured arteries that may bleed during surgical repair.

- The angiographic findings can affect the surgical approach. The surgical approach to complex acetabular fractures depends on the fracture pattern. Extensile exposures used in the open reduction of complex, displaced acetabular fractures requires the creation of a large abductor muscle flap using the superior gluteal artery as the foundation for the pedicle. Injury to the superior gluteal artery risks ischemic necrosis of the abductor muscles during extensile exposure because the ascending branches of the lateral femoral circumflex artery and the deep iliac circumflex arteries, which are the only major collateral circulation to the hip abductor muscles, must be divided.

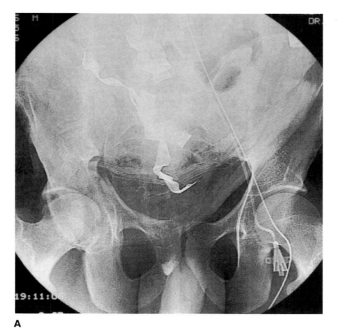

A

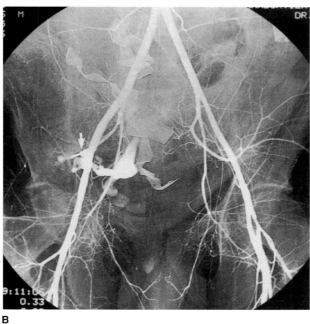

B

F I G U R E   1 1   24-year-old man involved in a motor-vehicle accident underwent immediate exploratory laporatomy for falling serial hematocrit values. An expanding retroperitoneal hematoma in the pelvis was noted, the abdomen was packed and patient immediately transported to angiography. **(A)** AP Pelvis Radiograph shows a complex right acetabular fracture with fragments displaced into the greater sciatic notch and widening of the right sacroiliac joint space. **(B)** Nonselective pelvic arteriogram performed via a left common femoral access shows brisk extravasation of contrast from the right superior gluteal artery *(arrow). (continued)*

Acetabular Fracture: Indications for Angiography (Continued)

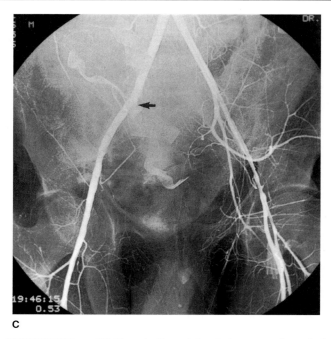

C

FIGURE 11 (CONTINUED)   (C) Nonselective pelvic arteriogram performed after embolization of the right internal iliac artery shows adequate stasis *(arrow)* and no other foci of active arterial hemorrhage.

Suggested Reading

Bosse MJ, Poka A, Reinert CM, Brumback RJ, Bathon H, Burgess AR. Preoperative angiographic assessment of the superior gluteal artery in acetabular fractures requiring extensile surgical exposures. *J Orthop Trauma.* 1988;2(4):303–307.

Intracapsular Femoral Neck Fracture

KEY FACTS

- Ninety-seven percent of intracapsular femoral neck fractures occur in patients over the age of 50; there is a strong association with diminished bone mineral.

- Patients usually sustain this fracture following a fall. The fall precedes the fracture in most cases, however, a fatigue fracture leading to a fall ("fracture and fall") can occur in severely osteopenic patients.

- Femoral neck fractures may involve the junction of the head and neck (subcapital), the mid portion (transcervical) or the base of the neck (basicervical). The subcapital fracture is more common in acute trauma whereas stress fractures are usually basicervical in location. Transcervical fractures are rare.

- Intracapsular femoral neck fractures are classified as:
  - Non-displaced
  - Displaced
  - Fatigue (or insufficiency)

- Complications of intracapsular femoral neck fractures include:
  - Osteonecrosis:
    - 10% to 15% in non-displaced or impacted fractures
    - 30% to 35% in displaced fractures
    - Nonunion
    - 25% to 33% in displaced fractures undergoing surgical reduction
    - Rare with non-displaced fractures
  - Displaced femoral neck fractures tend to compromise the blood supply to the femoral head. The major blood supply to the head is through the capsular vessels, not the vessels of the ligamentum teres. Other factors, such as an increase in intracapsular pressure leading to decreased venous return and diminished arterial perfusion, have also been implicated in compromising the blood supply to the femoral head.

Intracapsular Femoral Neck Fracture
(Continued)

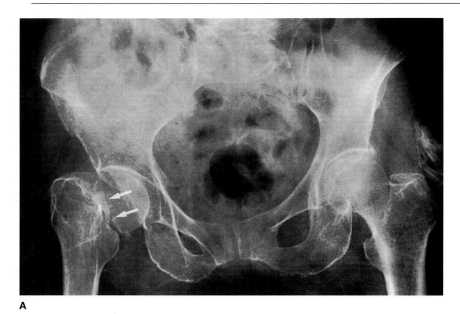

A

F I G U R E   1 2   **(A)** Case 1: AP digital radiograph of the pelvis shows a subcapital fracture of the right femoral neck *(arrows)*. The right femur is externally rotated: the lesser trochanter is clearly visible in profile and the greater trochanter overlaps the femoral neck, making its visualization more difficult, the usual situation in femoral neck fracture. The left hip is better positioned, but still not optimal. Best visualization of the femoral neck occurs when the hip is in internal rotation—the lesser trochanter is barely visible the greater trochanter is seen in profile.

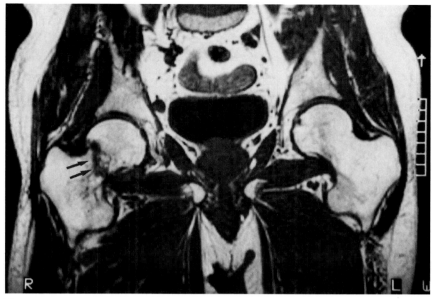

B

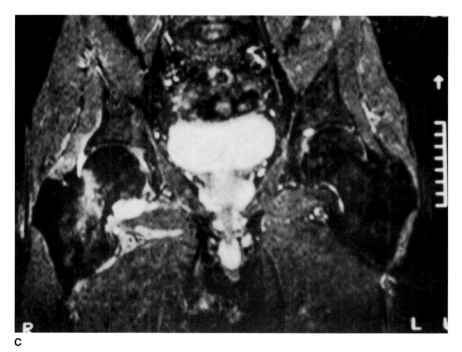

C

F I G U R E   1 2   Case 2: Occult hip fracture in an elderly lady with left hip pain following a fall. The plain films were normal. Coronal T1 **(B)** and STIR **(C)** images of the pelvis and hips show a linear band of low signal intensity on the T1 weighted images (*arrows,* B) in the femoral neck and a corresponding area of increased signal intensity on the STIR compatible with an occult subcapital hip fracture.

Suggested Reading

Swiontkowski MF. Intracapsular hip fractures. In: Browner BD, Jupiter JB, Levine AM, Trafton PG. ed. *Skeletal Trauma*. Philadelphia: WB Saunders; 1992:1369–1397.

Occult Hip Fracture

KEY FACTS

- The usual clinical setting for occult hip fracture is an elderly patient with hip pain following a fall.

- If good quality conventional radiographs are unrevealing, one still must rule out an occult femoral neck fracture. Occult intertrochanteric fractures are less common.

- Failure to recognize these injuries can lead to displacement and the complications of non-union or avascular necrosis. In the medically fragile patient, reduction with percutaneous pinning may greatly reduce morbidity, but can only be performed on non-displaced fractures.

- Diagnosis is often delayed when using conventional imaging strategies such as serial radiographs, tomography, and radionuclide bone scanning (RNBS). Such delays not only increase the incidence of displacement, which can occur at bed rest, but also increase morbidity in the elderly patient confined to bed.

- With RNBS there is substantial evidence that delays of 3 to 4 days are often necessary to maximize fracture detectability in elderly osteopenic patients.

- MRI can show the radiographically occult fracture within hours of the injury and is quite cost effective.

- Generally, T1 weighted coronal images and either T2 or STIR coronal images are obtained. The fracture is readily seen as a linear band of decreased signal intensity on T1 and increased signal intensity on T2 or STIR images.

- MRI can also detect other causes of occult hip pain, such as osteonecrosis, neoplasm, or pelvic fracture.

Suggested Reading

Rizzo PF, Lyden JP, Schneider RN. Occult hip fractures. *Contemp Orthop*. 1993;27(4): 339–345.

Stress-Insufficiency Fracture of the Femoral Neck

KEY FACTS

- Stress fractures can occur in younger, athletic patients or as insufficiency fractures in those with abnormal bone architecture or mineralization. The latter has also been implicated in elderly patients who fracture and fall (see Intracapsular Femoral Neck Fracture and Occult Hip Fracture).

- Stress fractures are more likely to occur in the lower aspect of the femoral neck above the intertrochanteric line (basicervical); subcapital fractures are more typical in the elderly patient who falls.

- The radiographic appearance is that of a band of sclerosis rather than a lucent line; the latter is seen when the fracture becomes complete. There can be some associated cortical thickening.

- Radiographs are initially normal in up to 40% of cases and can lag 2 to 6 weeks beyond the onset of symptoms.

- Under the appropriate clinical circumstances, MRI or radionuclide bone scan (RNBS) should be performed to facilitate early diagnosis and to prevent displacement of an occult fracture. If either study is normal, the diagnosis is for all practical purposes excluded. However, MRI is at least as sensitive as RNBS and when positive more specific.

- Femoral neck stress fractures are bilateral in approximately 10% of cases.

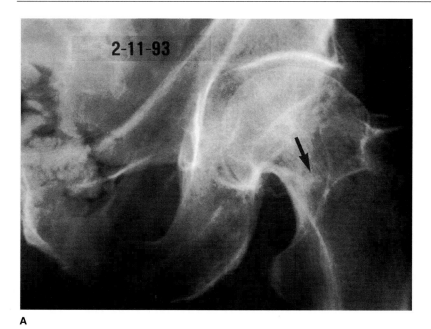

A

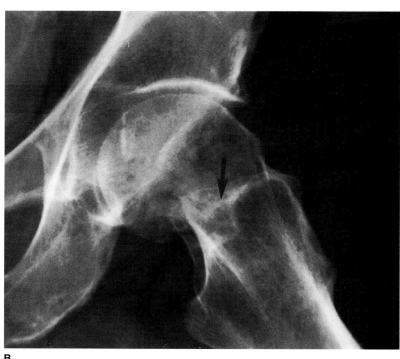

B

FIGURE 13   Elderly woman with left hip pain and no history of trauma or fall. **(A)–(C)** AP, lateral, and radionuclide bone scan. **(A)** and **(B)** AP view is externally rotated, a typical position for a patient in pain, making evaluation of the femoral neck difficult. However, there is a faint, linear zone of sclerosis seen near the base of the femoral neck *(arrows)*, that was seen only in retrospect, on the AP and lateral views **(A)** and **(B)**.

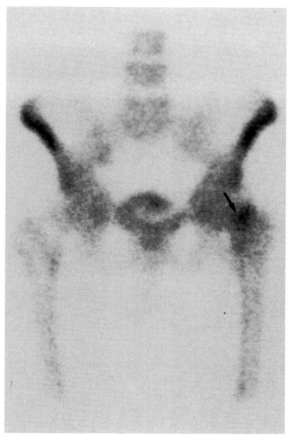

FIGURE 13

The bone scan demonstrates a linear band of increased activity *(arrow)* compatible with an occult, insufficiency fracture.

C

Suggested Reading

Keats TE. *Radiology of Musculoskeletal Stress Injury*. Chicago: Year Book Medical Publishers, Inc; 1990.

Intertrochanteric Femur Fracture

KEY FACTS

- Intertrochanteric femur fractures usually occur in the elderly patient, with women and men equally affected, unlike femoral neck fractures where the ratio is 3:1, respectively. Most of these fractures are due to falls, but are seen in younger patients suffering high energy traumatic injuries.

- Radiographs show that the main fracture line parallels the intertrochanteric ridge. The injuries are described in "parts," the four parts defined as the head/neck, shaft, greater and lesser trochanters.

- The incidence of the various intertrochanteric femur fractures types is as follows:

  - Two part: 25%

  - Three part: 35% (neck, shaft, lesser trochanter)

  - Four part: with varying comminution 40% to 50%

- Like femoral neck fractures, intertrochanteric femur fractures can be occult and MRI is used to detect these injuries (see Occult Hip Fracture).

  - In the setting of high energy trauma, up to 15% of these injuries can have an ipsilateral femoral shaft fracture

  - Non-union and osteonecrosis are rare in this fracture because of the abundant blood supply of the intertrochanteric region and the lack of injury to capsular vessels

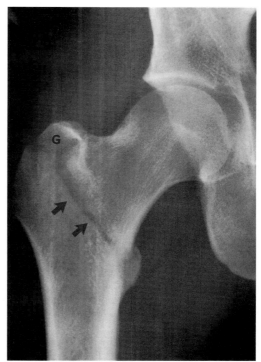

A

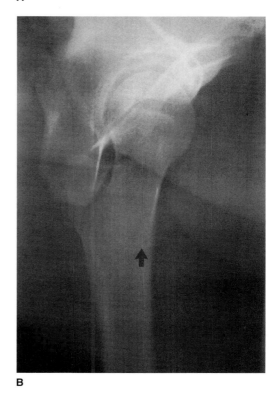

FIGURE 14

AP **(A)** and lateral **(B)** radiographs show a non-displaced fracture *(arrows)* along the intertrochanteric line with a separate greater trochanter (G) piece. Note that this fracture was in a patient in his mid-30s who sustained this injury in a motor-vehicle accident.

B

Suggested Reading

Rogers LF. *Radiology of Skeletal Trauma*. 2nd ed. New York: Churchill Livingstone; 1992: 1140–1148.

Subtrochanteric Femur Fracture

KEY FACTS

- While definitions vary, subtrochanteric femur fractures involve the area from the lesser trochanter to the proximal femoral diaphysis.

- Subtrochanteric femur fractures account for 10% to 34% of hip fractures and tend to occur in three populations:
  - Under 50 years—usually high energy trauma
  - Over 50 years—low energy trauma (i.e., falls)
  - Pathologic fractures

- Muscle attachments provide strong deforming forces that must be overcome during open or closed reduction and contribute to the incidence of non-union and malunion. Radiographs show:
  - Greater trochanter is adducted by gluteal muscles
  - Iliopsoas tendon flexes and externally rotates lesser trochanter
  - Femoral shaft is shortened and adducted by the hamstrings and adductors of the hip

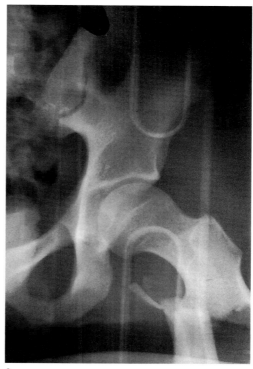

A

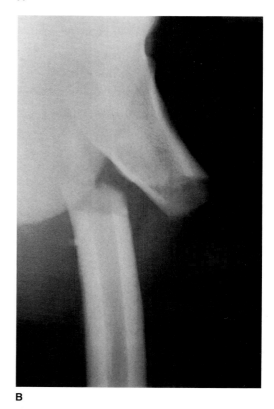

FIGURE 15

AP **(A)** and lateral **(B)** radiographs show a
typical subtrochanteric fracture of the left femur.
Note the abduction, internal rotation **(A)** and
flexion **(B)** of the femoral neck and trochanters.
There is also evidence of shortening and
adduction of the distal shaft fragment by the pull
of the adductors and hamstrings.

B

Suggested Reading

Russell TA, Taylor JC. Subtrochanteric fractures of the femur. In: Browner BD, Jupiter JB,
    Levine AM, Trafton PG. eds. *Skeletal Trauma*. Philadelphia: WB Saunders; 1992:
    1485–1524.

Femoral Shaft Fracture

KEY FACTS

- The femur is the longest, strongest, and heaviest bone in the body; therefore, it takes violent, high energy trauma to cause a fracture.

- Complications of the shaft fracture include significant blood loss (2 to 3 units) and venous thromboembolic complications in 40% to 90% of patients without appropriate prophylaxis.

- Femur fractures are usually seen in young adults as the result of vehicular accidents or gunshot wounds.

- Femur fractures are the most common long bone fracture in the multiply injured patient; up to 50% of such patients have ipsilateral femoral neck and tibial fractures.

- Approximately 15% are open fractures.

- Associated injuries with femur fractures include:
  - Neurovascular structures of the leg are usually spared except in supracondylar fractures and penetrating trauma (see supracondylar fracture)
  - Femoral neck, intertrochanteric fractures, and acetabular fractures
  - Associated tibial fracture leads to the "floating knee"
  - Knee ligamentous injury in 15%
  - CNS, visceral, chest and spine injuries often co-exist

- As a result of the associated fractures, radiographic evaluation of these patients must include the hip and tibia.

- Current treatment usually involves placement of an intramedullary nail (see Patella Fractures, Figure 17B).

Suggested Reading
Winquist RA, Hansen ST. Closed intramedullary nailing of femoral fractures: A report of five hundred and twenty cases. *J Bone Joint Surg.* 1984;66A:529–539.

Supracondylar Fracture of the Femur

KEY FACTS

- Supracondylar fractures are high energy injuries, the usual mechanism being direct trauma to the flexed knee, such as occurs when the knee violently strikes the dashboard during a motor-vehicle accident.

- Associated fractures include patella, femoral shaft or neck, and acetabulum as well as posterior hip dislocation.

- Popliteal vascular disruption has been reported in 10% to 40% of cases.

- Injury to soft tissue supporting structures of the knee are seen in up to 20% of patients and include cruciate and collateral ligaments, menisci, and capsular attachments.

- Typically the distal fragment is angled posteriorly due to the pull of the gastrocnemius.

- Extension into the knee joint is common with a vertical intercondylar component.

- Associated tibial shaft fracture may isolate the knee joint leading to the so-called "floating knee."

Supracondylar Fracture of the Femur
(Continued)

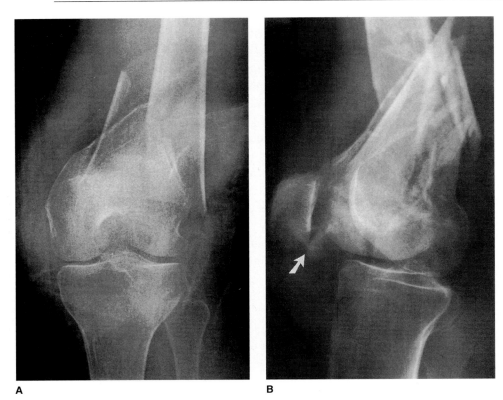

A   **B**

F I G U R E   1 6   AP **(A)** and lateral **(B)** views of the left knee show a comminuted supracondylar fracture of the distal femur. The lateral **(B)** shows typical angulation of the distal fragment as well as an avulsion off the lower pole of the patella *(arrow)*.

Suggested Reading

Benirschke SK, Swiontkowski MF. Knee. In: Hansen ST, Swiontkowski MF. ed. *Orthopaedic Trauma Protocols*. New York: Raven Press; 1993:291–293.

Patella Fracture

KEY FACTS

- Patellar fractures result from either direct blows or to tension stresses from the quadriceps muscle.

- Most fractures (60%) are mid-body and transverse; 25% are stellate or comminuted and 15% are vertical.

- Transverse fractures often require open reduction and internal fixation to overcome the tendency of the quadriceps muscles to distract the fracture.

- The knee striking the dashboard during a motor-vehicle accident is a frequent cause and may be associated with ipsilateral lower extremity, pelvic and acetabular injuries.

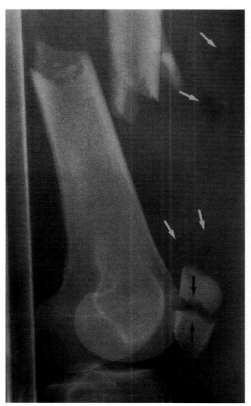 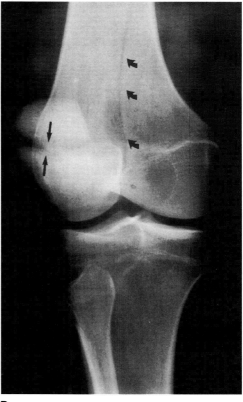

A   **B**

F I G U R E   1 7   Three patients with patellar fractures. Patient 1: **(A)** and **(B)**; Patient 2: **(C)**; Patient 3: **(D)** and **(E)**. **(A)** Lateral view of knee and distal femur shows a comminuted fracture of the junction of the middle and distal thirds of the femur, as well as a transverse fracture through the mid portion of the patella *(black arrows)*. Note the gas in the soft tissues *(white arrows)*—both fractures were open injuries. **(B)** The AP view shows the fracture of the patella *(black arrows)*, as well as a non-displaced fracture of the intercondylar region of the distal femur *(curved arrows).(continued)*

Patella Fracture (Continued)

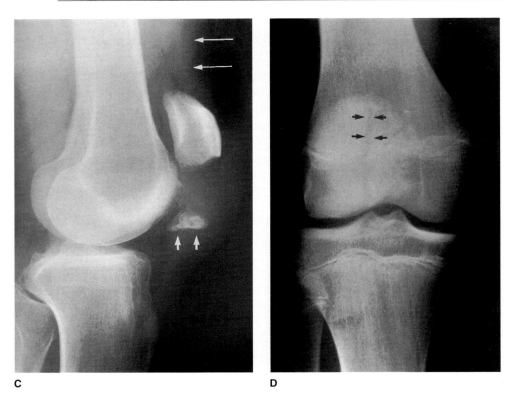

C   D

F I G U R E   1 7 (CONTINUED)   **(C)** The lateral radiograph of the knee shows avulsion of the inferior pole of the patella *(lower arrows)* with upward displacement of the upper pole and marked prepatellar edema. Note the wavy contour of the quadriceps tendon *(upper arrows),* indicating laxity due to the loss of the tethering effect of the patellar tendon attached to the distal fragment. **(D)** and **(E)** AP and patellar views of the knee show a non-displaced vertical fracture of the patella *(arrows).*

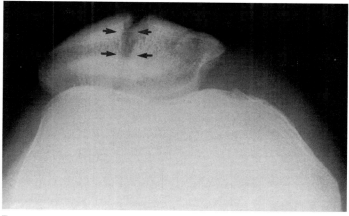

E

F I G U R E   1 7   See legend on facing page.

Suggested Reading

Rogers LF. *Radiology of Skeletal Trauma*. 2nd ed. New York: Churchill Livingstone; 1992: 1199–1284.

Tibial Plateau Fracture

KEY FACTS

- These fractures may involve lateral, medial, or both tibial plateaus, with extension into the metaphysis and diaphysis of the tibia in higher energy lesions.

- The usual mechanism of injury for a tibial plateau fracture is either a valgus stress and/or an axial load, creating a split, depression or combination of the two through the lateral tibial plateau.

- The cancellous trabeculae are stronger on the medial side of the knee joint because of its greater weight bearing load. Lateral injuries are, therefore, more common, accounting for 75% to 80% of cases of tibial plateau fracture.

- Isolated medial fractures are uncommon, reported in 5% to 10% of cases. Bicondylar injuries are seen in 10% to 15% of cases.

- Medial tibial plateau fractures are particularly severe, often with significant subluxation occurring at the knee joint. Like knee dislocations, they have a high incidence of neurovascular complications.

- A direct blow to the knee (e.g., being hit by a car) is seen in about 25% of cases; twisting falls and high-speed motor-vehicle accidents are also frequent causes.

- Compression fractures of the lateral plateau are usually seen in osteoporotic, older individuals and often have lower energy mechanisms.

- Ligamentous injuries are reported in 10% to 12% of tibial plateau fractures, with medial collateral ligament and anterior cruciate ligament injuries predominating.

- Radiographs show varying degrees of involvement of the plateau depending on the type of fracture. The goal of imaging these fractures is to show the number of fracture fragments, their displacement, and the degree of depression of the articular cortex. High resolution CT with sagittal and coronal reformations are utilized in most trauma centers. The use of MR is increasing in favor because of its ability to show not only osseous pathology, but also any associated internal derangement of soft tissue structures.

- Surgical indications include articular depression of more than 3 mm or varus or valgus instability of greater than 10°. These indications vary from center to center.

- Lateral meniscus pathology has been reported in up to 50% of cases, with meniscal displacement and lateral capsular instability commonly noted (Figure 18F).

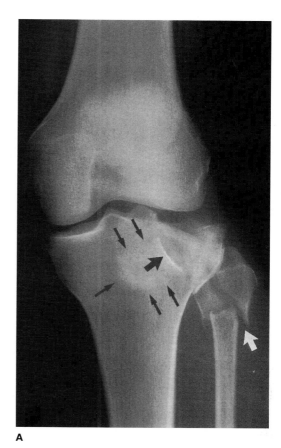

A

FIGURE 18

(A) AP radiograph of the knee shows a split depression type lateral tibial plateau fracture with comminuted fibular fracture *(white arrow)*. The articular cortex *(short black arrow)* is depressed and rotated with marked displacement of the associated metaphysis *(arrows,* also compare to D). **(B)** Cross table lateral of the knee shows a fat fluid level *(white arrows)*, a sign of intra-articular fracture; the depressed fracture is more subtle but visible on this view *(arrows). (continued)*

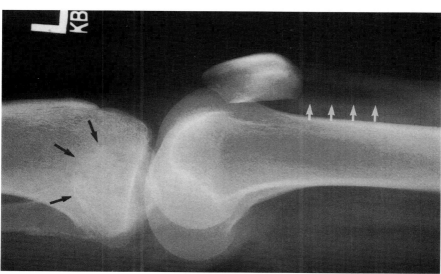

B

Tibial Plateau Fracture (Continued)

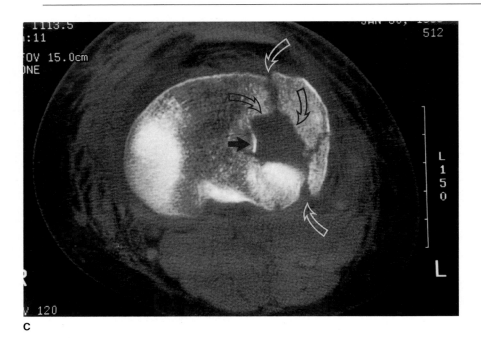

C

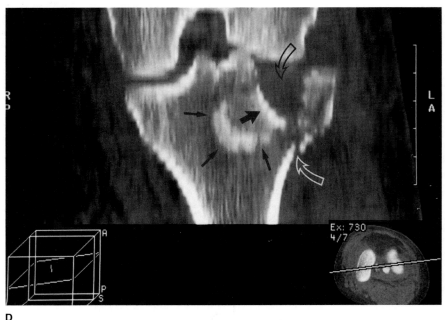

D

FIGURE 18 (CONTINUED)   High resolution axial CT **(C)** with coronal **(D)** and sagittal **(E)** reconstructions show the split *(open curved white arrows)* and the articular defect *(open curved black arrows)*in the lateral plateau in **(C)**. The degree of depression and rotation of the fragment are evident in **(D)** and **(E)**, respectively *(arrows)*.

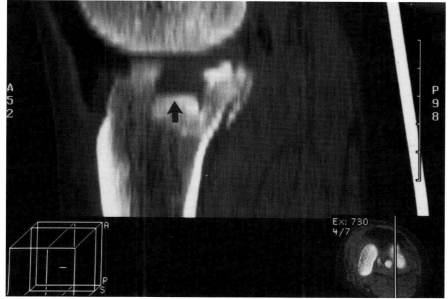

E

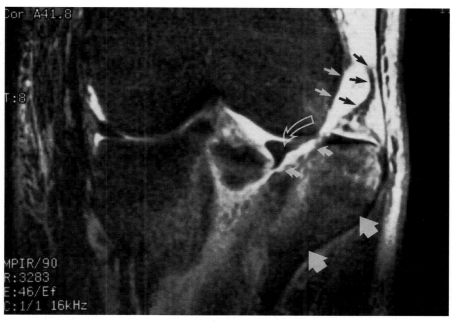

F

FIGURE 18   Another patient with tibial plateau fracture: Coronal STIR image **(F)** of the tibia in a patient with tibial plateau fracture. The image shows lateral displacement of the lateral plateau *(short, thick arrows)* and displacement of the lateral meniscus *(open white arrow)* into the fracture site *(small curved arrows)*, preventing reduction of the lateral condyle. The lateral capsule *(short black arrows)* is avulsed from the lateral femoral condyle *(short white arrows)* with intervening joint effusion.

Suggested Reading

Schatzker J. Tibial Plateau Fractures. In: Browner BD, Jupiter JB, Leving AM, Trafton PG. eds. *Skeletal Trauma*. Philadelphia: WB Saunders; 1992:1745–1757.

Tibial Spine (Anterior Cruciate) Avulsions

KEY FACTS

- True avulsions of bone occur at sites of ligamentous attachment.
- Avulsion of the anterior tibial spine usually occurs in children or adolescents, and is often associated with a fall from a bicycle.
- Radiographs show a bony fragment near the tibial spines anteriorly.
- The intact anterior cruciate ligament is attached to this fragment and if non-displaced may not require operation; with displacement, simple reattachment of the fragment may restore joint stability.
- In older individuals, the anterior cruciate ligament usually tears, requiring ligamentous reconstruction and carrying a far poorer prognosis than reattachment of an avulsed insertion.
- Differential diagnosis of avulsion of the anterior tibial spine includes other bony densities in the joint space, such as osteochondral fractures from the articular surfaces.

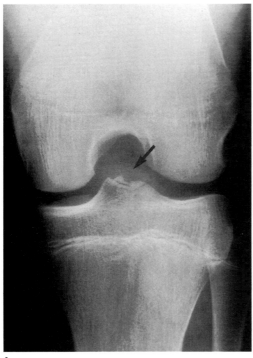 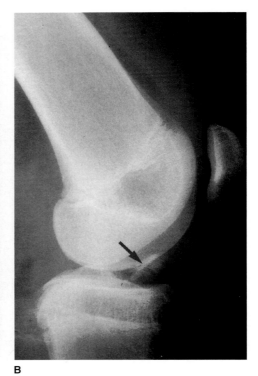

A   **B**

FIGURE 19   14-year-old boy who fell off his bicycle, complains of left knee pain and swelling. Frontal **(A)** and lateral **(B)** radiographs show a fragment of bone in the region of the tibial spines *(arrows)* consistent with an avulsion of the anterior cruciate ligament insertion. Sagittal proton density **(C)** and coronal STIR **(D)** images from an MR study confirm this impression. **(C)** Sagittal image demonstrates a large joint effusion *(open black arrow),* the ACL *(white, curved arrow)* attached to the avulsed fragment *(black arrow),* and the marrow edema at the site of avulsion in the tibial plateau. The proximal attachment of the ACL was normal on other images. **(D)** The coronal image shows the ACL *(curved arrow)* and the attached piece of tibial plateau *(white arrow).*

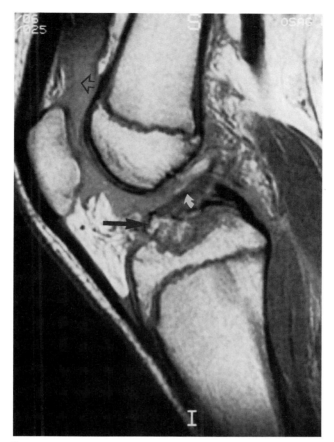

C

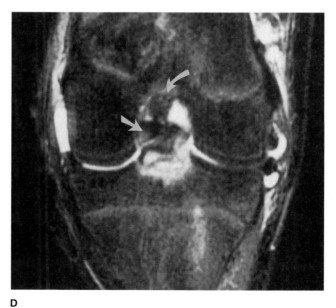

D

Suggested Reading

Baxter MP, Wiley JJ. Fractures of the tibial spine in children. *J Bone Joint Surg Br.* 1988;70:228.

Avulsion of the Posterior Cruciate Ligament Insertion

KEY FACTS

- The posterior cruciate ligament inserts on the posterior aspect of the tibial plateau.

- Avulsion of the posterior cruciate ligament insertion is usually the result of a knee striking the dashboard during a motor-vehicle accident forcing the tibia posteriorly, and is often associated with soft tissue injuries to the anterior aspect of the tibia. Athletic injuries resulting in a direct blow to the anterior tibia may produce this lesion as well.

- An avulsed bony fragment is commonly present over the posterior aspect of the tibial plateau on the lateral view.

- Other avulsions about the knee include:

    - The more common ACL avulsion

    - Lateral collateral ligament avulsions from either its origin or its insertion on the fibular head, in violent injuries such as knee dislocation

    - Medical-collateral ligament avulsions are rare, the ligament usually showing mid substance disruption

    - Avulsion at the insertion site of the posterior horn of the medial meniscus has been reported as well

    - Lateral capsular avulsions (see Segond Fracture: Lateral Capsular Avulsion)

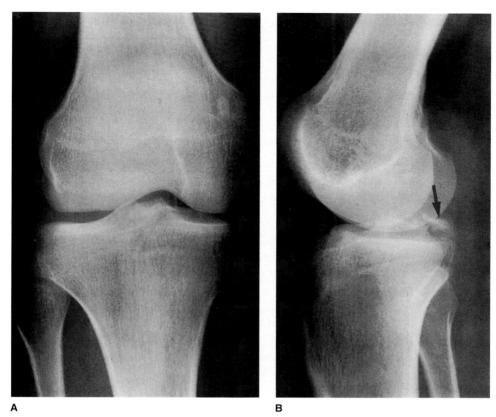

A   **B**

F I G U R E   2 0   24-year-old man involved as a passenger in an motor-vehicle accident; his anterior
tibia struck the dashboard and he complains of knee pain and swelling. AP **(A)** and lateral **(B)** radiographs
of the right knee. The AP view was unremarkable; the lateral shows an piece of posterior tibial plateau
(arrow) with the typical appearance of a posterior cruciate ligament avulsion.

Suggested Reading

Nagel DA, Burton DS, Manning J. The dashboard knee injury. *Clin Orthop.* 1977;126:
203–208.

The Unhappy Triad of O'Donoghue

KEY FACTS

- The Unhappy Triad of O'Donoghue was originally described as a combination of tears of the medial collateral (MCL), anterior cruciate (ACL) ligaments, and medial meniscus. With MRI scanning, there is a fourth component in most cases: bone contusions of the lateral femoral condyle and lateral tibial plateau, emphasizing the mechanism of injury.

- The mechanism of injury is a valgus stress with rotation, as in the clipping injury in football. The medial side of the joint is placed under tension, causing distraction of medial structures with compression of the lateral side of the knee.

- Involvement of the lateral rather than medial meniscus is common.

- A normal MCL shows continuity of the low signal ligament and no signal between the ligament and the overlying subcutaneous fat. MCL tears are classified as follows:
    - Grade I: sprain-normal continuity, abnormal signal intensity(SI)-increased SI on T2 or STIR, decreased SI on T1 weighted images. Function is usually preserved
    - Grade II: partial tear-abnormal SI in the soft tissues with distortion of the architecture of the ligament. Function compromised
    - Grade III: complete tear-loss of continuity of ligament, more extensive soft tissue SI abnormalities
    - The Grade II and III injuries can be difficult to distinguish on MRI scans

- The features of ACL tears are described in the next case, Anterior Cruciate Ligament Tear.

- Radiographs rarely show any significant abnormality except joint effusion.

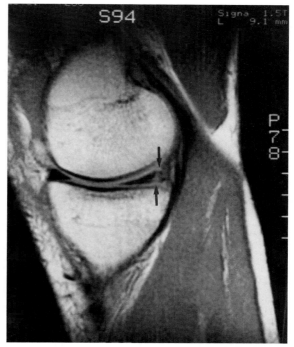

A

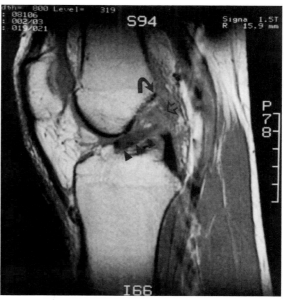

FIGURE 21

A 28-year-old male was playing touch football and sustained a clipping injury. MR examination of the right knee includes a sagittal proton density images through the medial aspect of the joint **(A)** and through the intercondylar notch**(B)** as well as a coronal STIR image **(C)** through the mid portion of the joint. **(A)** Grade III signal in the posterior horn of the medial meniscus *(arrows)* is seen. **(B)** The course of the ACL is abnormal *(arrowheads)* since it does not point toward the normal site of insertion *(curved black arrow);* the proximal part of the ACL is ill-defined *(open black arrow). (continued)*

B

The Unhappy Triad of O'Donoghue (Continued)

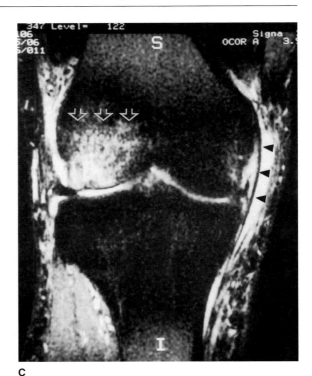

FIGURE 21 (CONTINUED)
(C) Coronal STIR image demonstrates an intact MCL *(black arrowheads)* surrounded by edema (bright signal surrounding ligament) and a bone contusion *(open white arrows)* of the lateral femoral condyle. Tears of the ACL and posterior horn of the medial meniscus were diagnosed and confirmed at arthroscopy. A partial tear of the MCL was diagnosed and confirmed clinically.

C

Suggested Reading
Mink JH, Reicher MA, Crues III JV, Deutsch AL. *MRI of the Knee*. New York: Raven Press; 1993.

Anterior Cruciate Ligament Tear

KEY FACTS

- The anterior cruciate ligament (ACL) originates from the posterior lateral aspect of the intercondylar notch of the femur and inserts anterior and medial to the anterior tibial spine. Its primary function is to prevent anterior translation of the tibia relative to the femur; it also resists hyperextension.

- On MR scans, the ACL should be taut and straight, forming a line clearly extending from origin to insertion. Signal within the ACL is common, often with 2 to 3 low signal intensity (SI) bands separated by higher SI tissue, presumably synovium or fat.

- The typical mechanism of injury involves external rotation of the femur on a fixed tibia with the knee in extension. Clipping injuries in football and skiing accidents are frequently involved activities.

- The ACL can tear in its proximal or distal aspect, but in most series, mid substance tears predominate. Partial tears are seen in up to one quarter of patients. Avulsions at the insertion are also seen [see Tibial Spine (Anterior Cruciate) Avulsions]. Complete and incomplete tears can be difficult to distinguish.

- Associated injuries include meniscal tears in up to 80% of cases (lateral, 66%; medial, 44%), medial collateral ligament and capsular disruptions, and osteochondral fractures. See also Segond Fracture: Lateral Capsular Avulsion and The Unhappy Triad of O' Donohough.

- MR findings of ACL tear include:
  - Large joint effusion with layering of blood products in the supine patient due to hemarthrosis
  - Loss of continuity and direction of ACL, with loss of straight line connecting origin and insertion
  - Waviness, with loss of taut appearance
  - Ill-defined mass replacing normal contours; a focal pseudomass may be seen at the site of the tear
  - Associated bone marrow edema is seen in up to 85% of ACL tears. One specific pattern with focal contusions of the anterolateral femoral and posterolateral tibial epiphyses is recognized and presumably occurs during the subluxation that accompanies these injuries
  - Anterior subluxation of the tibia relative to the femur-the "MR drawer sign"
  - Abnormal PCL contour ("buckling") often accompanies this subluxation

Anterior Cruciate Ligament Tear *(Continued)*

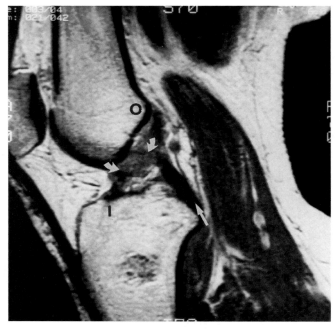

F I G U R E 2 2   Sagittal proton density image through the femoral notch demonstrates partial visualization of the distal part of the normal posterior cruciate ligament *(white arrow)*. There is a tear of the mid portion of the anterior cruciate ligament (ACL). A soft tissue mass *(curved white arrows)* interrupts the continuous line between the origin (O) and insertion (I) of the ACL.

Suggested Reading

Mink JH, Reicher MA, Crues III JV, Deutsch AL. *MRI of the Knee.* New York: Raven Press; 1993:141–162.

Meniscal Tears

KEY FACTS

- The normal meniscus is uniformly low in signal intensity on all MRI pulse sequences (Grade 0).

- Signal abnormalities of the menisci are graded as follows:
    - Grade I: globular or rounded signal focus within the meniscus, not communicating with a free intra-articular surface (i.e., the superior or inferior surfaces or free edge of the meniscus)
    - Grade II: linear signal within the meniscus, often extending to meniscocapsular junction but not involving a free surface
    - Grade III: linear signal that extends to a free intra-articular surface

- Significance of signal abnormalities:
    - Grade III signal on MR accurately predicts a mensical tear in over 90% of cases
    - Grade II signal has been shown to represent mucinous degeneration at pathologic correlation. These menisci may be symptomatic and most authors feel that such signal changes represent meniscal degeneration and/or intrasubstance tear
    - Grade I signal is generally asymptomatic and represents a lesser degree of mucinous degeneration at pathologic correlation

Meniscal Tears (Continued)

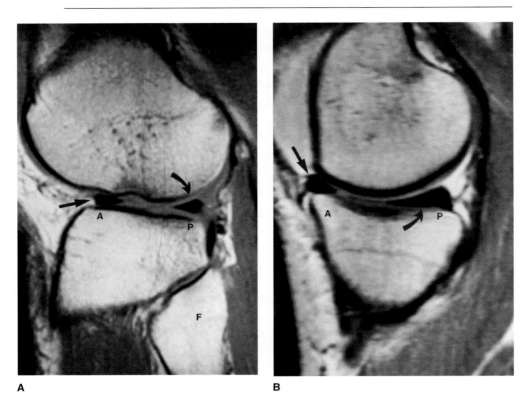

A   **B**

FIGURE 23   Grading System for Knee Menisci on MR. All images are from fast spin echo, sagittal proton density weighted sequences. Normal lateral meniscus (**A**) and medial meniscus (**B**) show homogeneous, low signal intensity (SI) and appear uniformly black. The posterior horn of the medial meniscus (*curved arrow*, B) should be larger than the anterior horn (*straight arrow*, B); in the lateral meniscus the posterior horn (*curved arrow*, A); and the anterior horn (*straight arrow*, A) are typically equal in size. (**C**) The globular increase in SI in the posterior horn of the medial meniscus *(curved arrow)* indicates grade 1 signal. (**D**). The linear increase in SI that does not communicate with a free articular surface *(curved arrow)* indicates grade 2 signal. (**E**) The linear zone of increased SI that communicates with the joint at the inferior aspect of the posterior horn of the medial meniscus *(curved arrow)* indicates grade 3 signal in a surgically proven tear. (**F**) The posterior horn of the medial meniscus is fragmented *(curved arrows);* linear areas of increased SI communicate with the superior and inferior surfaces to the meniscus. (A=anterior aspect of the tibial plateau; P = posterior aspect of the tibial plateau; F = fibula).

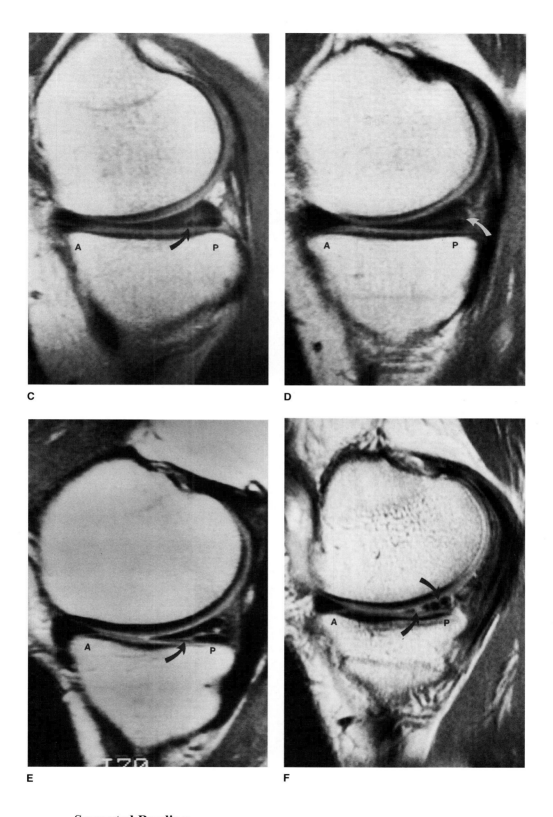

Suggested Reading

Stoller DW, Martin C, Crues JV, Kaplan L, Mink JH. Meniscal tears: Pathologic correlation with MR imaging. *Radiology*. 1987;163:731–35.

Segond Fracture: Lateral Capsular Avulsion

KEY FACTS

- Although often innocuous appearing on conventional knee radiographs, this avulsion represents a serious injury caused by forceful internal rotation with the knee in flexion.
- The lateral capsular ligament (a thickening of the lateral capsule at its mid portion) avulses a small piece of cortex of the tibia.
- This does not represent an avulsion of the lateral collateral ligament, which inserts on the fibular head.
- The Segond fracture is in the mid coronal plane and must be distinguished from the less common iliotibial band avulsion of Gerdy's tubercle more anteriorly on the tibia.
- Anterior cruciate ligament tears are reported in 75% to 100% of cases with meniscal tears noted in up to 70%.
- Radiographs show a small sliver of bone adjacent to the lateral tibial plateau near the joint line and a joint effusion.

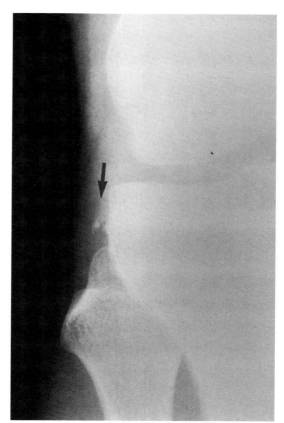

FIGURE 24

Close-up of the lateral side of the right knee joint **(A)** shows a small avulsion fracture *(arrow)* off the lateral side of the tibia, typical of Segond fracture. **(B)** Sagittal proton density MR image demonstrates lack of continuity of the ACL proximally *(arrow)* compatible with a tear.

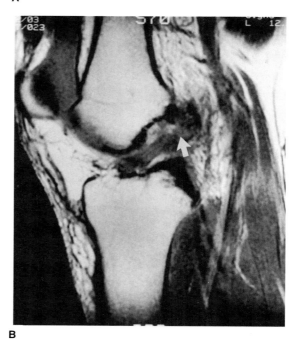

B

Suggested Reading

Goldman AB, Pavlov H, Rubenstein D. The Segond fracture of the proximal tibia: A small avulsion that reflects major ligamentous damage. *AJR*. 1988;151:1163.

Patellar Dislocation

KEY FACTS

- The patella normally sits in the trochlear sulcus of the anterior distal femur.

- Mechanism of injury in patellar dislocation usually involves internal rotation of the femur on a fixed foot, as in an abrupt change of direction in athletic activity.

- The patella usually relocates prior to clinical presentation. The patient often does not recognize the dislocation but offers a history such as "the knee gave out".

- The dislocation is almost always lateral, with disruption of the medial retinaculum. A tear of the vastas medialis obliquus muscle may also occur. The medial facet of the patella impacts upon the anterior lateral femoral condyle.

- The diagnosis may be uncertain in up to 50% of cases prior to MRI scanning. Patients may present clinically as anterior cruciate ligament tears or medial joint injuries.

- Radiographs are usually unremarkable except for a joint effusion.

- MR findings include:
  - Hemarthrosis in all patients
  - Disruption or sprain of medial retinaculum in 96%
  - Lateral patellar tilt or subluxation in 92%
  - Bone contusions, typically in lateral femoral condyle anteriorly (80%) and in the medial facet of the patella (20% to 40%)
  - Osteochondral injuries to the patella occur in 60%
  - Associated injuries to major ligaments or menisci in 30%

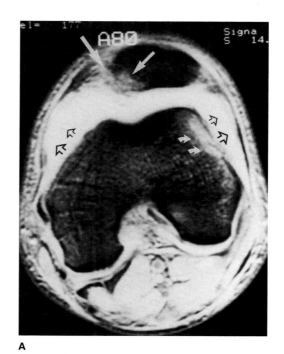

A

FIGURE 25

A 17-year-old woman complained that her knee "gave out" while playing soccer. Severe anteromedial knee pain and swelling followed. MR examination of the left knee includes axial gradient echo **(A)**, coronal T1 **(B)**, and STIR **(C)** pulse sequences. **(A)** Disruption of the attachment of the medial retinaculum to the patella *(white arrows)*, anterolateral femoral condyle contusion *(curved white arrows)* and large effusion *(open black arrows)* are noted. **(B)** Anterior coronal view at the level of the iliotibial band *(open arrows)* and Gerdy's tubercle *(curved black arrow)* shows the low intensity contusion/fracture in the lateral femoral condyle *(arrowheads)*. **(C)** Anterior coronal STIR image shows the high signal intensity marrow edema in the lateral femoral condyle *(white arrow)* and the large joint effusion *(open black arrows)*.

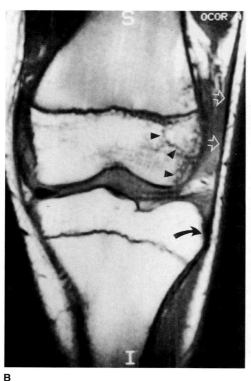

B

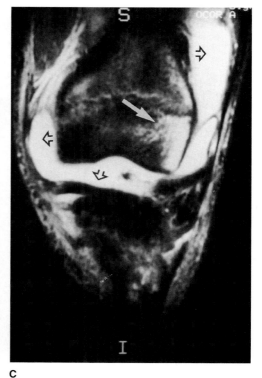

C

Suggested Reading

Kirsch MD, Fitzgerald SW, Friedman H, Rogers LF. Transient lateral patellar dislocation: diagnosis with MR imaging. *AJR*. 1993;161(1):109–113.

Knee Dislocation

KEY FACTS

- The classic definition of a knee dislocation involves clinical or radiographic evidence of displacement of the tibia relative to the femur.

- Using this definition, anterior and posterior dislocations account for 50% to 75% of cases. Medial, lateral, and rotational types also occur.

- Knee dislocations can go unrecognized because of spontaneous reduction during initial rescue or resuscitation; the marked laxity that results from extensive capsular and ligamentous injury appears to predispose to this spontaneous reduction.

- The mechanism of knee dislocation usually involves violent forces such as motor-vehicle accidents or falls from a significant height; multisystem traumatic injuries are often coexistent.

- Serious vascular injury to the popliteal vessels occurs in one third of cases and peroneal nerve injury in one fourth.

- The currently preferred definition is one of multidirectional instability of the knee due to a tear of the anterior cruciate ligament (ACL) plus combinations of posterior cruciate ligament (PCL), lateral collateral ligament (LCL), and medial collateral ligament (MCL) tears, as well as disruptions of capsular supporting structures.

- Radiographs may show gross displacement of the tibia relative to the femur, although minor degrees of suluxation or even normal alignment may be noted. The unstable knee in a patient with high energy trauma may be best evaluated with MRI. These patients often have associated injuries that make physical examination difficult or unreliable.

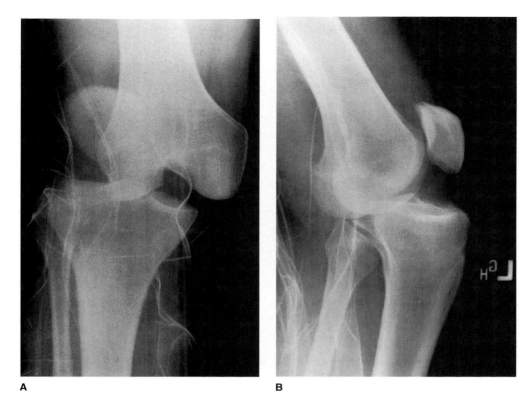

A   **B**

F I G U R E   2 6   AP **(A)** and lateral **(B)** views of the knee show anterior and lateral dislocation of the tibia and fibula on the femur. A pre-operative MR obtained 2 days later was obtained. *(continued)*

Knee Dislocation (Continued)

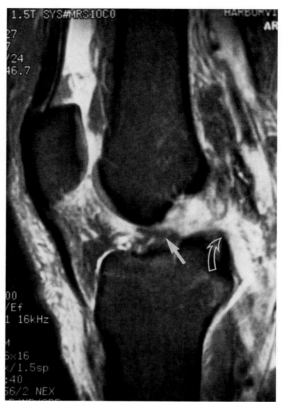

FIGURE 26 (CONTINUED)

A sagittal proton density image with fat suppression **(C)** shows a tear of the posterior cruciate ligament *(open white arrow)* and a tear of the anterior cruciate ligament (ACL)—the white arrow points to the remnant of the insertion of the ACL, with no visible ligament seen proximal. There is a suprapatellar bursal effusion and extensive edema anteriorly and posteriorly.

C

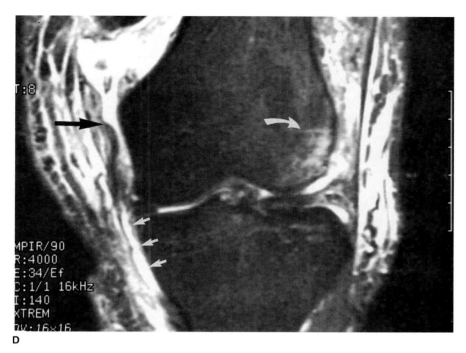

D

FIGURE 26   Coronal STIR **(D)** image shows an avulsion of the medial collateral ligament *(black arrow)* at its insertion, stripping of the medial capsule off the tibia *(white arrows)* and a bone contusion of the lateral femoral condyle *(curved white arrow)*. Extensive medial and lateral edema is noted. Both of these MR images are fat suppressed; the high signal (white) areas indicate either free fluid (i.e., suprapatellar bursa) or soft tissue edema.

Suggested Reading

Leffers D. Dislocations and soft tissue injuries of the knee. In: Browner BD, Jupiter JB, Levine AM, Trafton PG. eds. *Skeletal Trauma*. Philadelphia: WB Saunders; 1992:1724–1729.

Knee Dislocation and Arterial Injury

KEY FACTS

- Knee dislocations usually result from high-velocity injuries such as motor-vehicle accidents or falls from a significant height. Knee dislocations occur less frequently from low velocity mechanisms such as athletic injuries.

- The common classification of dislocation describes anterior, posterior, lateral, medial or rotatory displacements of the tibia relative to the femur. Anterior and posterior dislocations account for 50% to 75% of cases.

- The popliteal artery closely approximates the posterior aspect of the knee and is anatomically fixed both above and below the knee. Thus predisposing it to traumatic injury.

- Popliteal artery injury is seen in approximately one third of high-velocity knee dislocations and in 5% of low-velocity dislocations. Angiographic manifestation of arterial injury from a knee dislocation include spasm, non-occlusive narrowing (extrinsic compression by hematoma or intrinsic compression by mural hematoma), intimal flap, or abrupt/tapered occlusion. Angiographic demonstration of a pseudoaneurysm, arteriovenous fistula, and extraluminal contrast extravasation is extremely rare and usually associated with penetrating trauma.

- Our diagnostic algorithm is:
    - Threatened limb with loss of distal palpable pulses → immediate surgery
    - Diminished or non-palpable distal pulses in a viable limb and ankle-arm index >0.9 → conservative treatment
    - Diminished or non-palpable distal pulses in a viable limb and ankle-arm index <0.9 → angiography for depiction of type of arterial injury

- Spasm, non-occlusive narrowing and simple intimal flap are managed conservatively. All other forms of injury undergo surgical management.

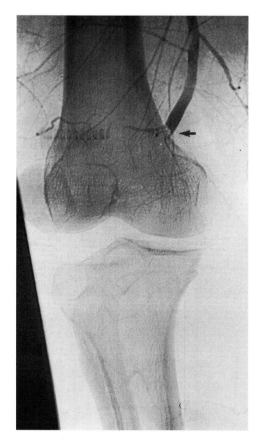

FIGURE 27

30-year-old woman sustained an anterior knee dislocation after a fall. Physical examination showed ligamentous instability of the knee and marked reduction in the ankle-brachial index. Angiography shows a sharp, abrupt occlusion of the proximal popliteal artery *(arrow)* and lateral joint space widening.

Knee Dislocation and Arterial Injury (Continued)

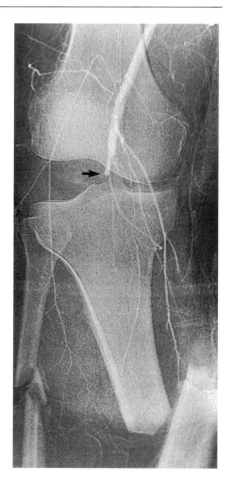

F I G U R E   2 8

40-year-old man, involved in a motorcycle accident, presented with displaced fractures of the tibia and fibula, instability of the knee joint and no palpable distal pulses. Angiography shows a tapered occlusion of the popliteal artery *(arrow)* at the knee joint.

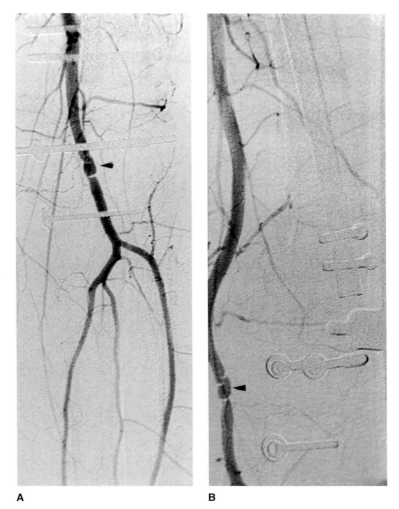

A   **B**

FIGURE 29   50-year-old man, involved in a motor-vehicle accident, sustained a comminuted fracture of the distal shaft of the femur. This was fixed by an intramedullary nailing with interlocking screws. Post-operatively, there was a decrease in the ankle-brachial index. AP **(A)** and lateral **(B)** angiographic views of the knee show intimal injury and irregularity of the below-the-knee popliteal artery segment *(arrowheads)*.

Suggested Reading

Kendall RW, Taylor DC, Salvian AJ, O'Brien PJ. The role of arteriography in assessing vascular injuries associated with dislocations of the knee. *J Trauma.* 1993; 35(6):875–8.

Tibial Stress Fracture

KEY FACTS

- The classic "runner's" stress fracture occurs in the proximal tibia.
- Radiographs show a zone of sclerosis with periosteal reaction and cortical thickening in the region of the posteromedial aspect of the proximal tibia.
- Stress fractures in the medial tibial plateau are also seen and can mimic internal derangement clinically.
- One must distinguish the terms "stress" and "insufficiency" fracture. The former involve abnormal stress on normal bone; the latter involve normal weight-bearing stresses on abnormal, usually osteoporotic bone.
- Anterior tibial stress lines are another form of reaction to chronic repetitive stress, usually in ballet dancers who repeatedly land on the plantar flexed foot. This mechanism creates a "bowstring" effect on the tibia, the gastrocnemius muscles placing the anterior cortex under tension. Short lucent lines in the anterior cortex, perpendicular to the long axis of the tibia are typical. This entity is sometimes confused with "shin splints"; the latter term is a clinical one referring to anterior tibial pain.
- Radiographic findings can lag behind symptoms by 2 to 6 weeks. MRI scanning or radionuclide bone scanning can expedite the diagnosis.
- Failure to recognize a stress fracture can lead to complete fracture, as in this case.

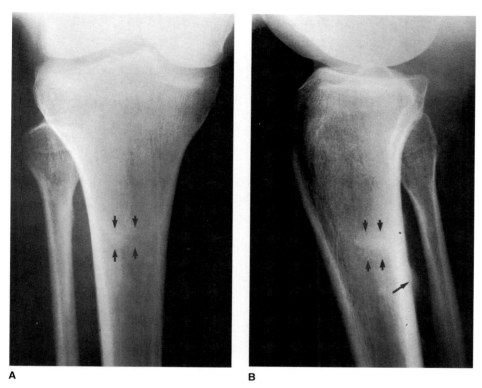

A   **B**

F I G U R E   3 0   Case 1: Tibial stress fracture converted into a complete fracture. Knee pain in a 23 year-old graduate student who had been running to get in shape for her upcoming ski trip. AP **(A)** and lateral **(B)** radiographs at time of original presentation show a linear zone of sclerosis in the proximal tibia posteromedially (*short arrows,* A and B). Some posterior periosteal thickening is noted **(B)** *(arrow).* *(continued)*

Tibial Stress Fracture (Continued)

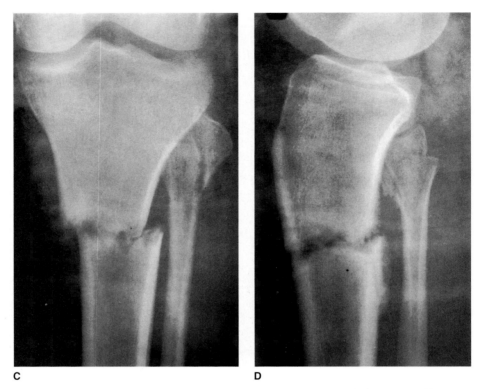

C   D

F I G U R E   3 0   (CONTINUED)   Despite warnings to the contrary, she decided to go skiing and
presented to a local emergency room following a fall on her first run on the slopes. Transverse fractures
were noted on anterior and lateral **(C)** and **(D)** films of the tibia in the same location as the sclerosis noted
in **(A)** and **(B).**

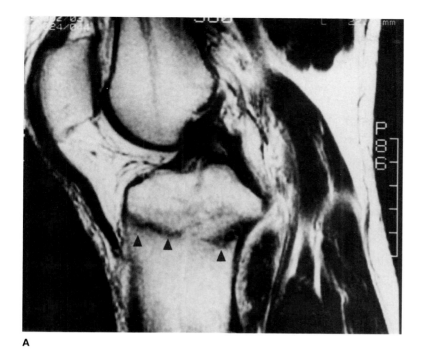

A

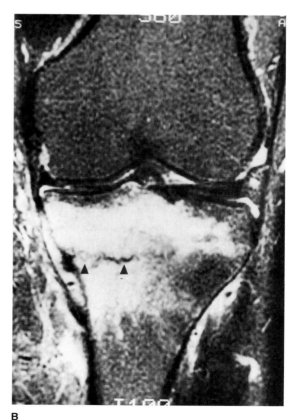

B

FIGURE 31

Figures **(A)** and **(B)** are MR scans in another runner with proximal tibia pain and equivocal radiographs. The sagittal proton density **(A)** and coronal STIR images **(B)** demonstrate a linear, low intensity (i.e., black) focus in the tibial metaphysis *(arrowheads)* consistent with a fracture. The surrounding high (white) signal in **(B)** represents bone marrow edema. This stress fracture was more proximal than usual and presented clinically as a possible meniscal tear.

Suggested Reading

Keats TE. *Radiology of Musculoskeletal Stress Injury*. Chicago: Year Book Medical Publishers, Inc; 1990.

Tibial and Fibular Shaft Fractures

KEY FACTS

- Fractures of the tibial and fibular shafts are classified by anatomic location, pattern of fracture lines, and number of fragments.

- As a general rule, AP and lateral views are sufficient to diagnose and characterize these fractures.

- The radiographic findings are rarely subtle, even in nondisplaced fractures.

- As with the forearm, the tibia, fibula, and the proximal and distal tibiofibular joints represent a fibro-osseous ring. Fractures involving both bones are unstable, while isolated tibial or fibular shaft fractures are stable.

- Proximal fibular shaft fractures and fibular neck fractures can be associated with injuries to the ankle mortise.

- Whenever an isolated injury to one bone is seen, careful clinical and radiologic assessment of the ankle joint and proximal tibio-fibular joint should be made.

- In small children, nondisplaced spiral fractures (toddler's fractures) of the tibial shaft may be difficult to see on some views. Two perpendicular plane, good quality, radiographs are therefore essential.

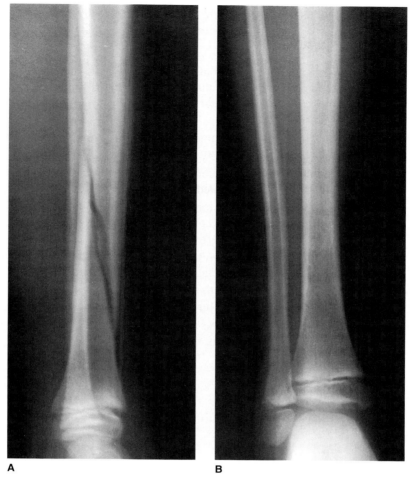

A   **B**

F I G U R E   3 2   Toddler's fracture. The spiral tibial shaft fracture is shown well on **(A)** the lateral view, but is almost invisible on **(B)** the AP view. No fibular fracture was detected in this child.

Suggested Reading

Russell TA, Taylor JC, LaVelle DG. In: Rockwood CA, Green DP, Bucholz RW. eds. *Rockwood and Green's Fractures*. Philadelphia: Lippincott; 1991:1915–1982.

Rogers LF. In: *Radiology of Skeletal Trauma*. New York: Churchill Livingstone; 1992: 1284–1301.

Tibial Plafond Fracture (Pilon Fracture)

KEY FACTS

- Supramalleolar fractures of the distal tibia that extend into the tibial plafond are known as Pilon fractures. They are usually associated with fractures of the distal fibula and/or disruption of the distal tibiofibular syndesmosis.

- These fractures are a combination of injuries to the ankle and the distal tibial metadiaphysis, usually with intra-articular comminution.

- The mechanism of injury is vertical loading (e.g., jumpers). The forces drive the talus upward through the tibial plafond.

- The compressive nature of the force usually results in articular cartilage damage and outcomes are often poor, in spite of anatomic reductions. Persistent pain and early osteoarthritis are common.

- Almost all of these injuries require internal fixation and they frequently present a major surgical challenge to the orthopaedist.

- For the radiologist the most important things to identify are the extent and severity of the tibial plafond injury.

- Standard AP, lateral, and mortise views of the ankle are adequate for initial evaluation. CT scan is useful for preoperative planning.

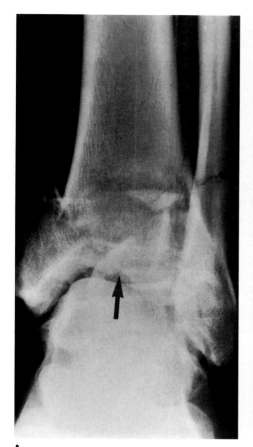

A

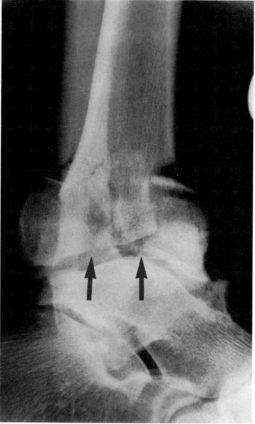

B

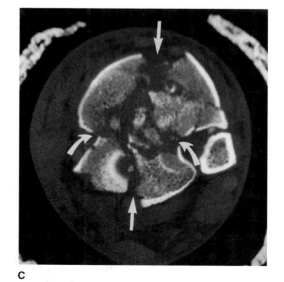

C

F I G U R E   3 3

This patient sustained a severely comminuted tibial plafond and distal fibular fractures by falling from a third floor window. The AP **(A)** and lateral radiographs **(B)** show the comminuted tibial fracture, extending into the articular surface *(arrows)*. **(C)** A CT scan clearly shows the sagittal *(arrows)* and coronal *(curved arrows)* components of the fracture. *(continued)*

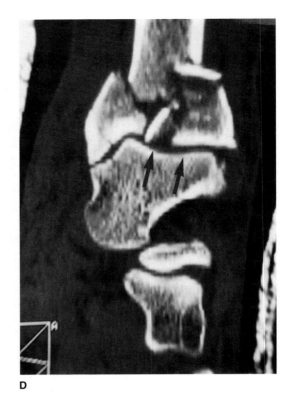

D

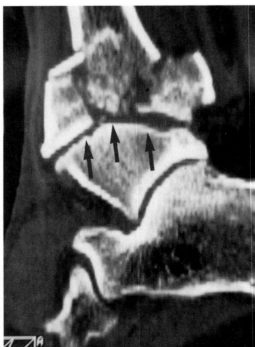

FIGURE 33 (CONTINUED)
Reconstructions in the coronal (**D**) and sagittal
planes (**E**) show how the talar dome *(arrows)*
has been forced proximally, through the distal
tibia, with displacement of tibial fragments away
from the center of the plafond.

E

Suggested Reading

Rogers LF. In: *Radiology of Skeletal Trauma*. New York: Churchill Livingstone; 1992:1382–1385.

Vander Griend RA, Savoie FH, Hughes JL. In: Rockwood CA, Green DP, Bucholz RW. eds.
Rockwood and Green's Fractures. Philadelphia: Lippincott; 1991:1983–2033.

Ankle Mortise Injuries: Classification

KEY FACTS

- There are two popular classification systems for fractures involving the ankle mortise. These are the Danis-Weber classification and the Lauge-Hansen classification.

- The Danis-Weber classification classifies ankle fractures according to the position of the fibular fracture (if one is present) relative to the distal tibiofibular syndesmosis. Type A is below, type B through, and type C above the syndesmosis.

- For orthopaedists planning surgery, the Danis-Weber scheme is very useful, however, it often does not help the radiologist predict coexisting ligament injuries.

- The Lauge-Hansen classification is based on extensive studies of mechanisms of injury and catalogs the sequence of events.

- Because the Lauge-Hansen scheme follows the sequence of events, it helps predict ligamentous injuries. This enables us to be more accurate in diagnosis, and to select additional investigations more appropriately. It is therefore an important classification for radiologists to understand.

- Four basic mechanisms exist in the Lauge-Hansen classification. Each is named according to the position of the foot and the time of injury and the direction of motion of the talus, relative to the ankle mortise: Supination-Adduction, Pronation-Abduction, Supination-External Rotation and Pronation-External Rotation. Each of these four mechanisms is associated with a characteristic fibular fracture (Figures 28 to 32).

- Whichever classification is used, the most important consideration is ankle stability. A single break in the fibro-osseous ring of the ankle mortise is stable. Two or more breaks will render the ankle unstable. Unstable fractures usually need operative fixation.

- Whenever instability is suspected but not demonstrated, stress radiographs of the ankle should be performed.

Ankle Mortise Injuries: Classification
(Continued)

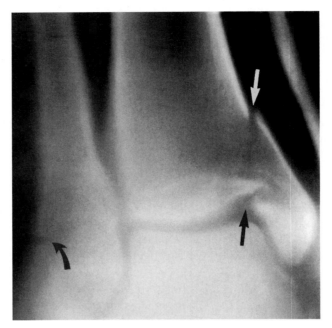

FIGURE 34   AP tomograph of a supination-adduction injury. There are two stages to this injury. In stage one, the direct pull on the lateral malleolus produces a transverse fracture *(curved arrow)*. In stage two, the direct push on the medial malleolus produces a vertical fracture at the junction of the malleolus and the plafond *(straight arrows)*.

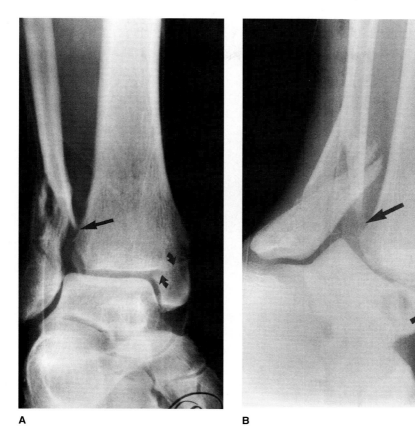

A   B

FIGURE 35 AP views of two different patients with typical pronation-abduction injury. There are three stages to this injury. In stage one, the pull on the medial malleolus produces a fracture that is usually transverse. In stage two, the push on the lateral malleolus ruptures the tibiofibular syndesmosis. In stage three, the distal fibula is bent laterally and fractures immediately above the syndesmosis. This final stage is a fracture of the fibula, immediately above the syndesmosis, known as the bending fracture. In both of the cases shown here, the transverse medial malleolar fracture *(curved arrows)* is displaced, the talus is shifted laterally and the syndesmosis is wide. In both patients, the bending fracture of the fibula shows its characteristic spike of bone *(straight arrows)* pointing directly at the upper margin of the tibio-fibular syndesmosis. The presence of this spike is the most reliable method for recognizing a pronation-abduction injury.

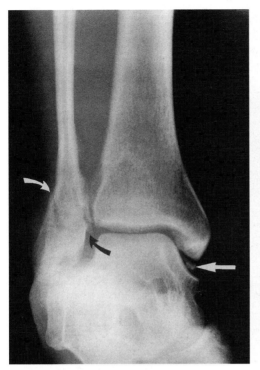

A

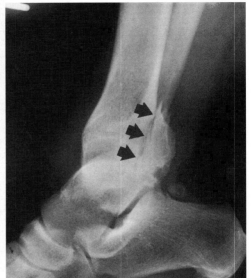

B

FIGURE 36

(A) AP and (B) lateral views of a typical
supination-external rotation injury. There are four
stages to this injury. The initial force pulls down
on and twists the lateral malleolus outward. Stage
one is a rupture of the anterior tibiofibular
ligament. Stage two is a spiral lateral malleolar
fracture *(curved arrows)*. Stage three is a posterior
malleolar fracture *(short, broad arrows)* or
posterior tibiofibular ligament rupture. Stage four
is a medial malleolar fracture *(long straight
arrow)*. In this patient, the medial malleolar
fracture is a small fragment, representing avulsion
of the deltoid ligament. In (C) another patient, the
entire medial malleolus has been avulsed *(long
straight arrow),* with displacement of the lateral
malleolar fragment *(curved arrows)* and marked
lateral talar shift.

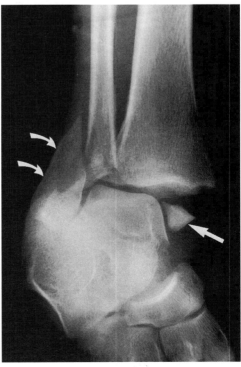

C

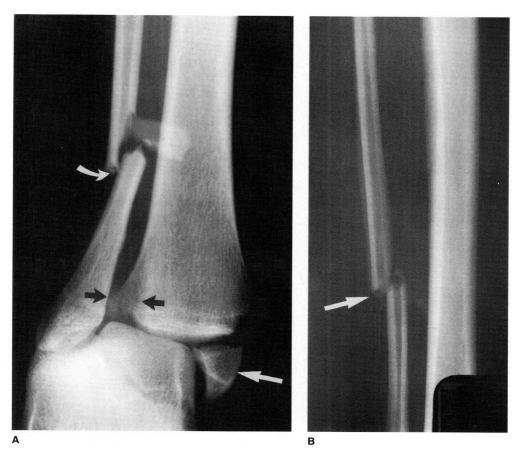

A   **B**

F I G U R E   3 7   **(A)** AP view of a typical pronation external rotation injury. There are four stages to this injury. The initial force pulls down on the medial malleolus, twisting it outward. Stage one is a medial malleolar fracture *(long arrow)*. Stage two is an anterior tibiofibular ligament rupture and tear of the distal interosseous membrane. Stage three is a fracture through the distal fibular shaft one to two inches above the syndesmosis. The fibular fracture is usually oblique and is often comminuted *(curved arrow)*. Stage four is a posterior malleolar fracture or posterior tibiofibular ligament rupture. Note the syndesmosis widening *(short arrows)* and lateral talar shift. **(B)** In some patients the fibular shaft fracture *(arrow)* may be farther up the leg and will not be seen on a routine ankle film. A high fibular fracture should be suspected in any patient with talar shift and no fibular fracture visible on the ankle films.

Ankle Mortise Injuries: Classification
(Continued)

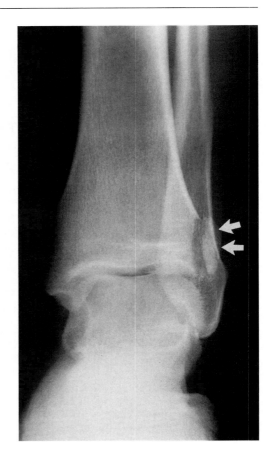

FIGURE 38

Avulsion of the anterior tubercle of the tibia *(arrows)* can occur in external rotation injuries as an alternative to rupture of the anterior tibio-fibular ligament. This is known as the Tillaux-Chaput fracture. Similar avulsions of the anterior tubercle of the fibular can also occur. These injuries can be isolated, as in the case shown here, or associated with the other characteristic fractures and dislocations of external rotation injuries. Isolated injuries, such as this are usually stable and do not normally require fixation.

Suggested Reading

Rogers LF. In: *Radiology of Skeletal Trauma*. New York: Churchill Livingstone; 1992: 1319–1382.

Vander Griend RA, Savoie FH, Hughes JL. In: Rockwood CA, Green DP, Bucholz RW. eds. *Rockwood and Green's Fractures*. Philadelphia: Lippincott; 1991:1983–2033.

Cuneiform Fracture

KEY FACTS

- Isolated cuneiform injuries are uncommon. If fractures of these bones are present, a more serious injury involving the adjacent bones and joints should be suspected.

- Subtle cuneiform injuries can be overlooked with standard foot radiographs.

- Reverse oblique views are helpful for profiling the medial cuneiform.

- If surgical repair is planned, CT scan is helpful for reliably defining fracture extent and severity.

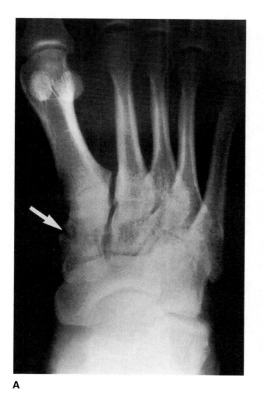 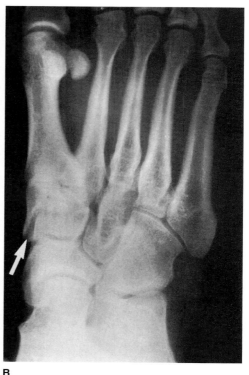

A   **B**

FIGURE 39

Medial cuneiform fracture. This minimally displaced fracture *(arrows)* is visible on both **(A)** AP and **(B)** oblique views but could not be seen on the lateral view. *(continued)*

Cuneiform Fracture (Continued)

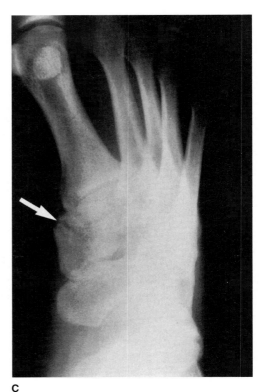

F I G U R E   3 9   (CONTINUED)
It is best shown, however, on **(C)** a reverse oblique
view.

C

Suggested Reading

Rogers LF. In: *Radiology of Skeletal Trauma*. New York: Churchill Livingstone; 1992:1433–1443.
Heckman JD. In Rockwood CA, Green DP, Bucholz RW. eds. *Rockwood and Green's Fractures*. Philadelphia: Lippincott; 1991:2139–2140.

Calcaneal Fracture

KEY FACTS

- The calcaneus is the most commonly fractured bone of the adult foot (60%). The injury is intra-articular in 75% and extraarticular in 25% of adults; in children, the fractures are usually extra-articular.

- The usual mechanism involves a fall onto the heel, often off a ladder or roof.

- Associated injuries include:
  - Ipsilateral lower extremity fracture in 20% to 46%
  - Spine fractures in 10% to 30%
  - Peroneal tendon entrapment in the lateral wall fracture

- Extra-articular fractures include fractures of the tuberosity, Achilles avulsions (in children and in some diabetic adults), and anterior process avulsions.

- Intra-articular fractures include joint depression and tongue-type injuries. Both involve the posterior facet of the subtalar joint, but the latter has a horizontal fracture line that exits through the dorsum of the tuberosity below the Achilles tendon insertion. This tongue fragment contains the posterior facet of the subtalar joint, which can be displaced by the pull of the Achilles tendon. In the more common joint depression injury, the posterior facet is separated from the tuberosity.

- Intra-articular fractures result from an axial load, which drives the lateral process of the talus into the underlying calcaneus, creating three fracture fragments: the tuberosity, lateral fragment containing one half to two thirds of the posterior facet, and the sustentaculum tali, including middle facet and remaining part of the posterior facet. The fracture often extends into the calcaneocuboid joint. Injury to the talus is rare.

Calcaneal Fracture *(Continued)*

FIGURE 40

Bilateral intra-articular calcaneal and L1 compression fractures: Films on a patient who fell 20 feet off a wet roof. Lateral radiographs of the right **(A)** and left **(B)** calcaneus show bilateral calcaneal fractures. **(A)** A joint depression fracture *(straight arrows)* is present with loss of Boehler's angle and depression of the posterior facet of the subtalar joint *(curved arrows)*. The middle facet is shown by the black arrows. **(B)** A tongue type fracture is present; the tongue fragment extends to the posterior margin of the calcaneal tuberosity *(white arrow)* and includes the posterior facet of the subtalar joint *(curved arrows)*, necessitating surgical reduction and fixation to prevent displacement by the pull of the Achilles tendon.

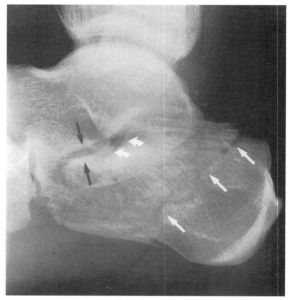

A

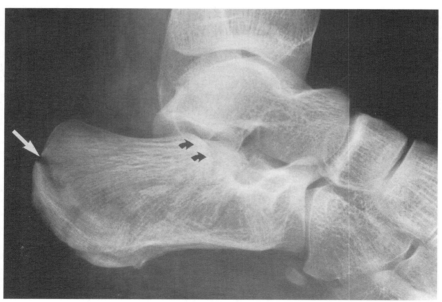

B

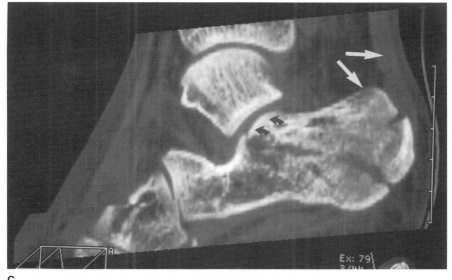

C

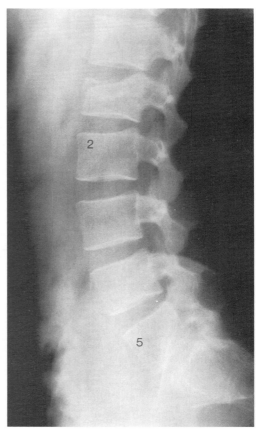

FIGURE 40

(C) High resolution CT reformation, sagittal plane demonstrating the tongue fragment and the Achilles tendon *(straight arrows)* and the posterior facet *(curved arrows).* (D) Lateral lumbar spine radiograph shows a compression fracture of L1.

D

Calcaneal Fracture (Continued)

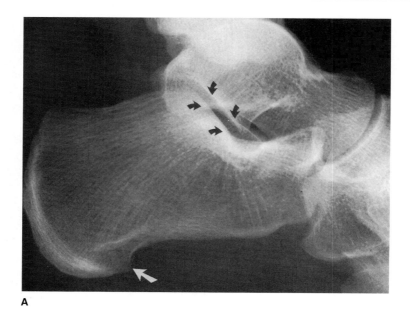

A

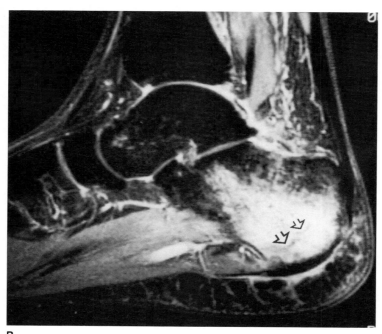

B

FIGURE 41   Occult calcaneal fracture: A lateral radiograph **(A)** of the calcaneus demonstrates a subtle break in the cortex *(arrow)*. The posterior facet of the subtalar joint *(curved arrows)* is normal and can be compared to Figure 39 **(A)** and **(B).** A sagittal STIR MR **(B)** scan shows extensive marrow edema in the calcaneus (the bright signal-compare to the normal talus or navicular) and a fracture line *(open arrows)* extending into the tuberosity.

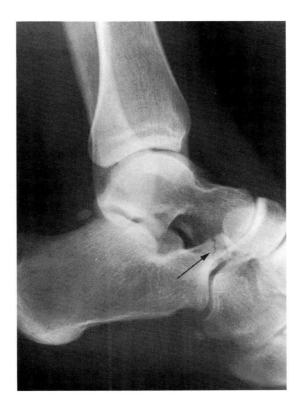

FIGURE 42

Anterior process fracture: A lateral radiograph of the ankle shows an avulsion of the anterior process of the calcaneus *(arrow)*.

Suggested Reading

Rogers LF. *Radiology of Skeletal Trauma*. 2nd ed. New York: Churchill Livingstone; 1992:1443–1463.

Talus Fracture

KEY FACTS

- Articular cartilage covers 60% of the talus; in addition, there are no muscle or tendon insertions. As a result the blood supply is tenuous.

- The main arterial supply to the talus enters laterally via the tarsal tunnel, near the inferior margin of the neck. It supplies part of the neck of the talus and most of the body.

- Fractures through the neck of the talus can compromise the blood supply in a manner analogous to scaphoid waist fracture, leaving the body of the talus at risk for osteonecrosis (ON).

- Mechanism of injury usually involves abrupt dorsiflexion of the foot with delivery of high energy forces as in vehicular accidents or falls.

- Associated injuries include ipsilateral fractures of foot and ankle in 16% of patients. Approximately one quarter of patients will have fractures elsewhere, reflecting the high energy nature of the injury.

- Approximately one half of fractures of the body and neck involve subtalar dislocation or posterior talar dislocation from the ankle mortise.

- Most orthopaedic surgeons use the Hawkins classification, which describes the injuries in terms of displacement of the fractures and associated joint dislocations. It is useful in predicting the likelihood of ON.
  - I: Non-displaced vertical fractures-incidence of ON less than 10 %
  - II: Fractures with subtalar subluxation or dislocation- incidence of ON of 40%
  - III: Fracture with tibiotalar and subtalar dislocation-ON in over 90%
  - IV: Features of type III with extrusion of the body, often through an open wound and talonavicular dislocation-ON in nearly 100%

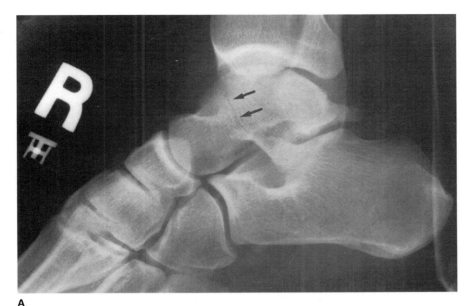

F I G U R E   4 3   **(A)** and **(B)** Patient 1: Non-displaced fracture of the body of the talus *(arrows)* is seen on a lateral radiograph **(A)** and sagittal reconstruction **(B)** from a high resolution CT scan (1 mm slice thickness).

Talus Fracture (Continued)

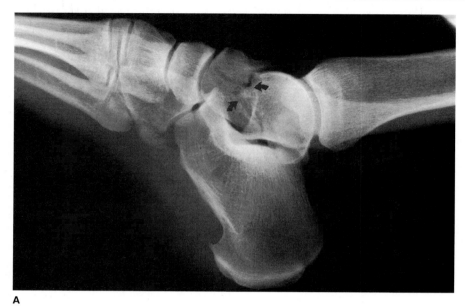

A

B

F I G U R E   4 4   Patient 2: A lateral radiograph **(A)** and a sagittal reconstruction **(B)** from a high resolution CT show a fracture of the neck of the talus *(arrows)*.

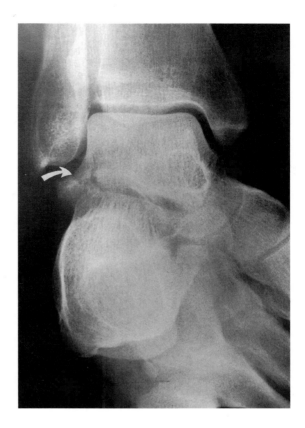

FIGURE 45

Patient 3: Mortise (oblique) view of the ankle shows a non-displaced fracture of the lateral process of the talus *(arrow)*. Fractures of this region may mimic routine ankle sprains or fractures clinically and can be missed if not sought.

Suggested Reading

Hansen ST. Foot injuries. In: Browner BD, Jupiter JB, Levine AM, Trafton PG. eds. *Skeletal Trauma*. Philadelphia: WB Saunders; 1992: 1959–1991.

Talar and Subtalar Dislocations

KEY FACTS

- Most dislocations are associated with talar fracture.
- Pure subtalar dislocation without fracture requires simultaneous dislocation of the talonavicular joint. Total talar dislocation is rare and includes the tibiotalar joint.
- Subtalar dislocations are distributed as follows: medial (56%); lateral (34%); posterior (6%); anterior (4%).
- Medial subtalar dislocations are the result of an inversion force with the calcaneus and navicular lying medial to the talus with an intact ankle mortise.
- Lateral subtalar dislocations result from eversion forces, with the navicular and calcaneus lateral to the talus.
- Associated osteochondral injuries are common; CT should be considered in all such dislocations to detect any loose bodies in the subtalar or talonavicular joints. At times an entrapped fragment can prevent anatomic reduction.
- Subluxations are more subtle and may involve only the subtalar joint. Careful examination of the alignment of the posterior facet of the subtalar joint on the lateral radiograph and the relationship of the talus to the calcaneus on the AP radiograph are essential in making the diagnosis.

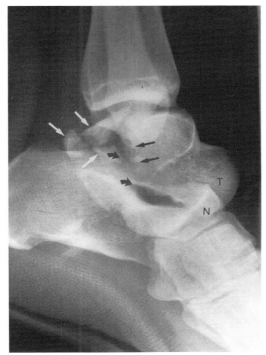

A

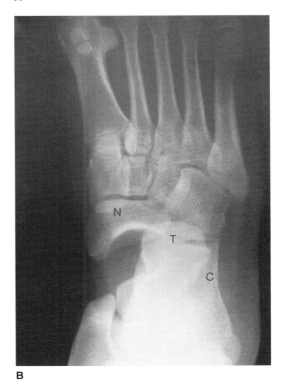

B

FIGURE 46

(A) Lateral radiograph of the hindfoot shows a
fracture dislocation of the talus at the subtalar
joint and a talonavicular dislocation. Films
show fracture into the subtalar articular surface
(straight black arrows) with comminuted
pieces of the posterior talus *(white arrows)* and
the normal calcaneal side of the posterior facet
of the subtalar joint *(curved black arrows).* **(B)**
AP radiograph of the foot shows medial
dislocation with the navicular (N) and
calcaneus **(C)** displaced medial to the talus
(T); the tibiotalar joint is intact. There is a
fiberglass posterior splint in place.

Suggested Reading

Berquist TH, Johnson KA. Trauma. In: Berquist TH. ed. *Radiology of the Foot and Ankle*. New
York: Raven Press; 1989:174–175.

Tarsal Navicular Fracture

KEY FACTS

- Three types of tarsal navicular fracture occur: avulsion, tuberosity, and body.

- Capsular avulsions at the dorsal margin at the talonavicular joint are common and account for about half of navicular fractures.

- The medial aspect of the navicular is the tuberosity; it serves as site of insertion for the posterior tibial tendon. Avulsion of the tuberosity may occur with forced eversion or abduction of the foot (see the next case, "The Nutcracker Fracture of the Cuboid").

- Fractures of the body of the navicular are often associated with midfoot fracture-dislocation and account for about one fourth of navicular fractures.

- Both horizontal and vertical fracture patterns are noted in the body of the navicular. Displacement of fragments is common in these injuries.

- The talonavicular subtalar and tibiotalar joints are essential joints for normal biomechanical function of the foot. Anatomic restoration following navicular body fracture often requires surgical stabilization.

- Stress fractures and non-displaced body fractures can be difficult to detect on conventional radiographs. With a clinical suspicion of occult navicular injury, MRI scanning would be the procedure of choice. High resolution CT scanning in multiple planes is an alternative.

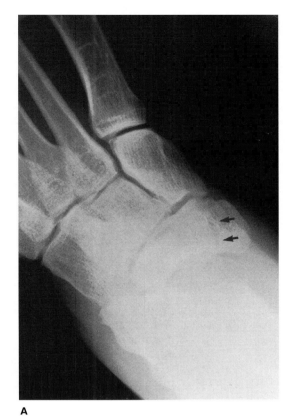

A

FIGURE 47

AP **(A)** and lateral **(B)** views of the foot show a subtle fracture line *(arrows)* through the navicular. *(continued)*

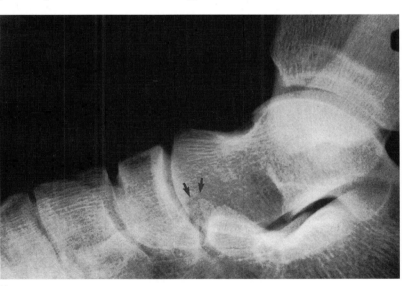

B

Tarsal Navicular Fracture (Continued)

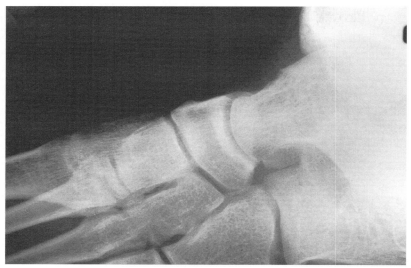

C

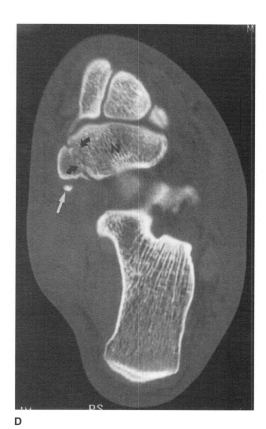

F I G U R E   4 7 (CONTINUED)

An oblique view **(C)** did not show the fracture, but it was confirmed on high resolution CT (*curved arrows,* D). The density proximal to the navicular in **(D)** *(white arrow)* proved to be an accessory ossicle. These fractures can be quite subtle and often require additional radiographs or CT as in this case. (N = navicular).

D

Suggested Reading

Sangeorzan BJ, Benirschke SK, Mosca V et al. Displaced intra-articular fractures of the tarsal navicular. *J Bone Joint Surg Am.* 1989;71:1504.

The Nutcracker Fracture of the Cuboid

KEY FACTS

- Cuboid fracture due to *indirect* compressive forces is designated the "Nutcracker" fracture.

- This fracture occurs when abduction of the forefoot compresses the cuboid between the bases of the fourth and fifth metatarsals distally and the calcaneus proximally "like a nut in a nutcracker".

- These fractures are significant clinically because they can interfere with the mechanical alignment of the foot or involve displacement of articular surfaces.

- The valgus stress typically crushes the cuboid articular surface and may avulse the insertion of the posterior tibialis tendon on the navicular medially. Other compressive injuries may involve the calcaneus or bases of the fourth and fifth metatarsals.

- Fractures secondary to direct trauma or associated with dislocation, stress fractures, and toddler's fractures have also been reported. Fractures of the cuboid are uncommon injuries with avulsion fractures of the cuboid most frequently encountered.

- Avulsions are usually periarticular, proximally at the calcaneocuboid joints or distally in association with Lisfranc injuries.

The Nutcracker Fracture of the Cuboid
(Continued)

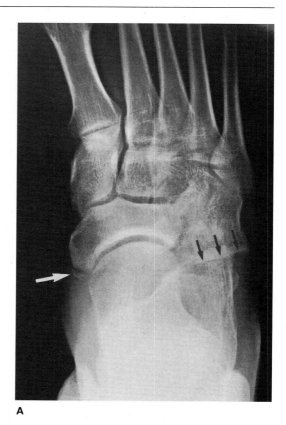

A

FIGURE 48

AP **(A)** radiograph of the foot shows poor definition of the calcaneocuboid joint *(black arrows)* as well as an avulsion of the insertion of the posterior tibialis tendon medially off the navicular *(white arrow)*. The lateral **(B)** film shows a fracture of the body *(curved arrow)* and compression of the articular surface of the cuboid *(arrows)*.

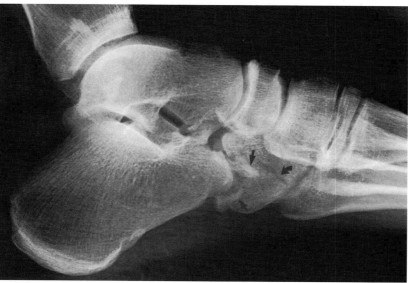

B

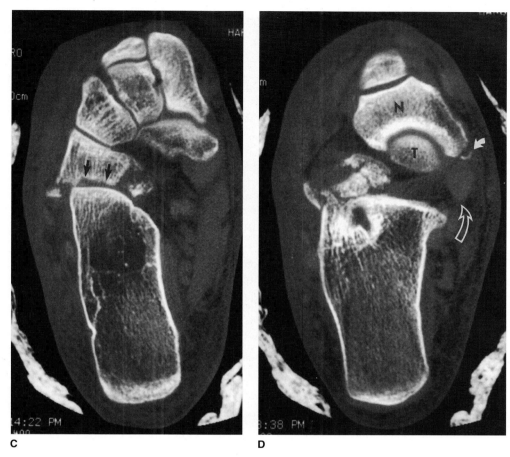

C   **D**

F I G U R E 4 8   This is further highlighted by the axial high resolution CT (1 mm slices, 1 mm intervals) (*arrows* in **C**). Axial CT through the talonavicular (T, N) joint in (**D**) demonstrate the avulsion fracture *(curved arrow)* and the distal posterior tibialis tendon *(open white arrow).*

Suggested Reading

Hermel MB, Gershon-Cohen J. The nutcracker fracture of the cuboid by indirect violence. *Radiol.* 1953;60:850–854.

Tarsometatarsal (Lisfranc's) Fracture Dislocation

KEY FACTS

- The tarsometatarsal (TMT) joints are known as the Lisfranc's joints. Injuries typically involve their stabilizing ligaments with or without associated fracture.

- The mechanism of tarsometatarsal fracture dislocation is usually involves forced plantar flexion. The "bunk bed fracture" in children is an example.

- The transverse metatarsal ligaments span the metatarsal (MT) bases II to V; the medial aspect of the II MT is attached to the medial cuneiform by an oblique ligament, but not to the first MT.

- The middle cuneiform is shorter than the medial and lateral bones, creating a mortise or recess for the base of the second metatarsal, locking the latter between the surrounding tarsal bones.

- This unique osseous and ligamentous anatomy predisposes to separation of the I and II MT under high stress. Higher energy injuries result in even greater degrees of disruption and involvement of more metatarsals.

- Fracture patterns of tarsometatarsal fracture dislocation include:

  - Divergent (I MT medial, II to V lateral)

  - Homolateral (all MTs shift lateral)

- The plantar ligaments and tendons provide more support than the dorsal soft tissues and, therefore, dorsal displacement is more common.

- Imaging includes AP, lateral, and medial oblique views of the foot. Stress views are used to diagnose purely ligamentous lesions. Comparison radiographs are useful for subtle ligamentous injury. CT scanning can detect subtle chip fractures. Bone scanning or MRI scanning can be used to detect occult injuries, although physical examination and stress views under anesthesia usually suffice.

- On stress views of the symptomatic and normal sides displacement or distraction of the involved tarsometatarsal joint by greater than 2 mm is an indication for surgical stabilization. These surgical indications vary fom center to center.

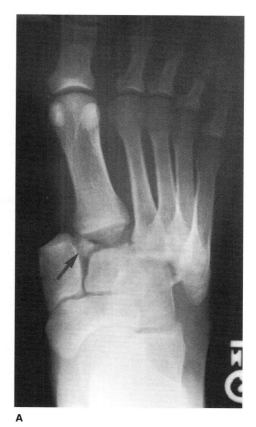

F I G U R E   4 9

Case 1: AP **(A)** and lateral **(B)** views of the foot
show a homolateral Lisfranc's fracture dislocation.
(A) Lateral subluxation of all of the metatarsals is
typical of the homolateral pattern. The small bony
fragment *(arrow)* has avulsed from the base of the
second metatarsal at the site of attachment of the
ligament to the medial cuneiform. **(B)** The lateral
view looks unremarkable at first glance, but note
the lack of normally visualized TMT joints *(arrows)*
as the only evidence of the injury.

A

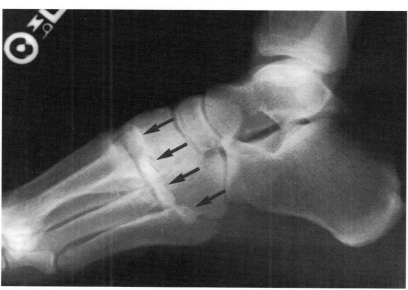

B

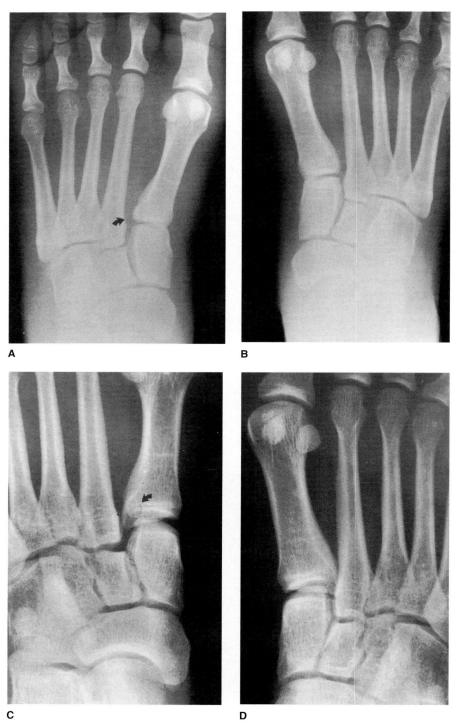

FIGURE 50   Case 2: AP radiographs of the left **(A)** and right **(B)** foot show subtle widening of the space between the first and second metatarsals (*arrow,* Figure 48A). Valgus stress views under anesthesia of the left **(C)** and right **(D)** foot show the instability at the TMT joints on the right indicative of a Lisfranc's ligamentous injury. A non displaced fracture of the base of the I MT was also seen (*arrow* in A).

Suggested Reading

Hansen ST. Foot injuries. In: Browner BD, Jupiter JB, Levine AM, Trafton PG, eds. *Skeletal Trauma*. Philadelphia: WB Saunders; 1992:1959–1991.

Metatarsal Fracture

KEY FACTS

- Direct injury is the most common mechanism of metatarsal fracture. Typically, a heavy object falls on the foot.
- Indirect forces can be applied by twisting injuries, resulting in spiral fractures of the metatarsal shafts, particularly the first three.
- Twisting injuries can also result in avulsions of tendon or ligament insertions. The most common of these occurs at the base of the fifth metatarsal—the insertion of peroneus brevis. The term "Jones fracture" should be confined to transverse fractures of the fifth metatarsal base, within 1.5 cm of the tuberosity.
- Fifth metatarsal base fractures are usually classified as intra-articular or extra-articular. While most of these fractures are treated conservatively, the presence of intra-articular deformity makes surgical fixation an option.
- Anteroposterior, oblique, and lateral radiographs are usually adequate to characterize metatarsal fractures.

Metatarsal Fracture (*Continued*)

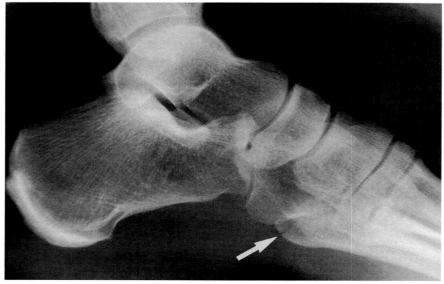

A

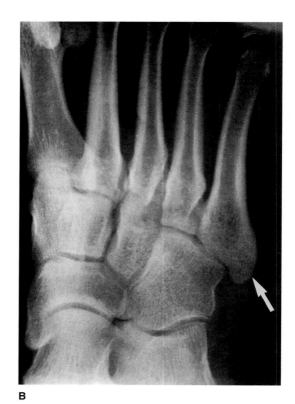

B

FIGURE 51

Intra-articular fifth metatarsal base fracture. Often misinterpreted clinically as ankle injuries, these fractures *(arrows)* are often visible on lateral views of the ankle. In this patient the non-displaced fracture is much easier to see on (**A**) the lateral view of the ankle than on (**B**) the oblique view of the foot.

Suggested Reading

Rogers LF. In: *Radiology of Skeletal Trauma*. New York: Churchill Livingstone; 1992: 1498–1516.

Heckman JD. In: Rockwood CA, Green DP, Bucholz RW. *Rockwood and Green's Fractures*. Philadelphia: Lippincott; 1991: 2151–2166.

Toe Injuries

KEY FACTS

- Injuries to the toes usually result from direct blows. Either objects are dropped on the unprotected foot or the toe is stubbed against a hard object.

- Most great toe fractures are minimally displaced.

- Lesser toe fractures will often involve multiple toes and are frequently displaced, angulated, or rotated.

- The interphalangeal or metatarsophalangeal joints are often involved in toe fractures.

- Dislocations of the metatarsophalangeal or interphalangeal joints occur when axial loads are applied to the toes. These dislocations are most commonly dorsal.

- AP, lateral, and oblique radiographs of the affected toes are usually sufficient to evaluate these fractures and dislocations.

- Foreign bodies are common in the toes and feet, particularly in countries where shoes are not worn routinely. In the USA, many of these injuries occur indoors, walking barefoot and stepping on hidden objects in carpet. Radiographs are essential in the initial workup of all foreign bodies. While wood and plastic are frequently invisible on radiographs, metal and glass are readily demonstrated.

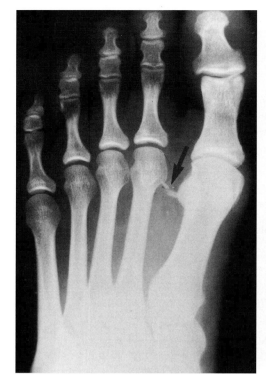

A

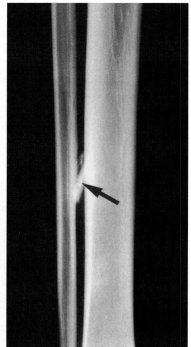

B

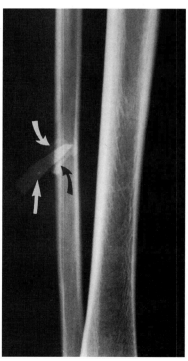

C

FIGURE 52

Foreign bodies in foot and leg. **(A)** This patient
cut the sole of his foot on a broken window. The
densities *(arrow)* between the heads of the first
and second metatarsals are pieces of glass. Glass
has a similar density to calcium on radiographs.
All patients who are cut by glass should have the
area radiographed. **(B)** AP and **(C)** lateral views of
another patient demonstrate a large piece of glass
(arrows) in the soft tissues adjacent to the fibular
shaft, that has been present for 3 weeks. The
laceration had been sutured at the time of injury
and radiographs were not obtained. The patient
presented 3 weeks post injury with a wound
infection. Note the periosteal new bone *(curved
arrows* in C) surrounding the foreign body.

Suggested Reading

deLacey G, Evans R, Sandin B. Penetrating injuries: How easy is it to see glass (and plastic)
    on radiographs? *Br J Radiol*. 1985:58;27–30.

Subject Index

Note: Page numbers in *italics* refer to illustrations, *t* following page numbers indicates tables.